Dear Robert + Barb

You two do so much for
Credo and Nashville. Thanks for all
your help.

Paul

NASHVILLE MEDICINE

A History

JAMES SUMMERVILLE

Foreword by U.S. Senator William H. Frist, M.D.

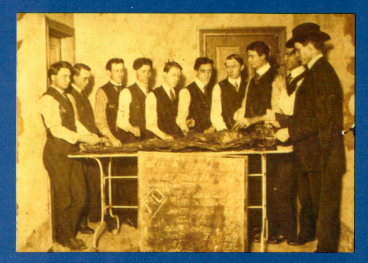

1900s

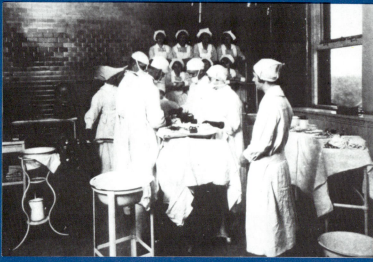

1920s

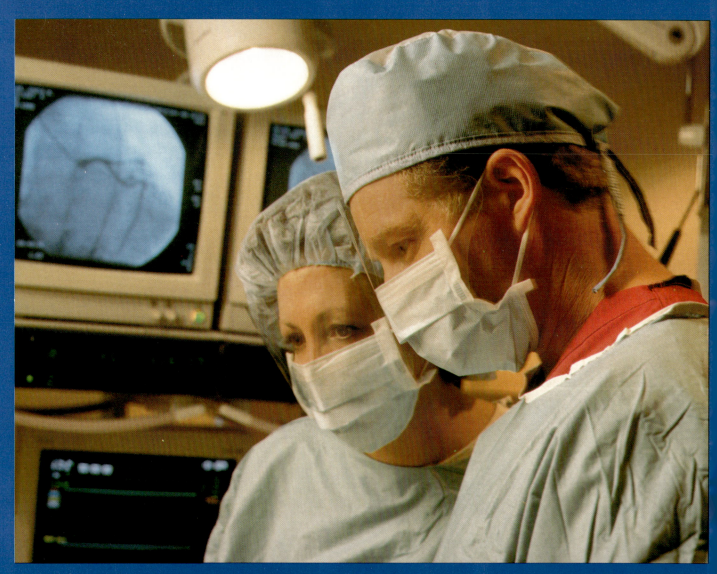

1990s

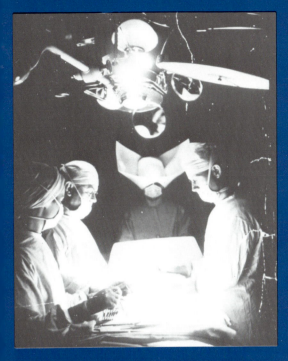

1940s

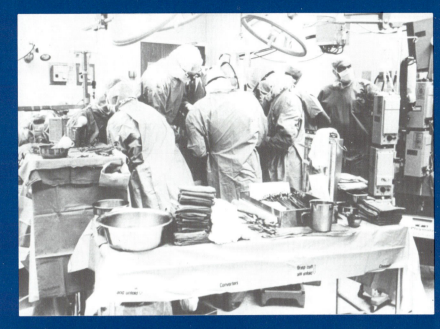

1960s

NASHVILLE MEDICINE
A History

JAMES SUMMERVILLE

Foreword by U.S. Senator William H. Frist, M.D.

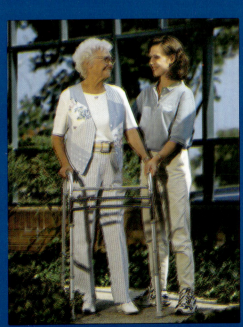

1990s

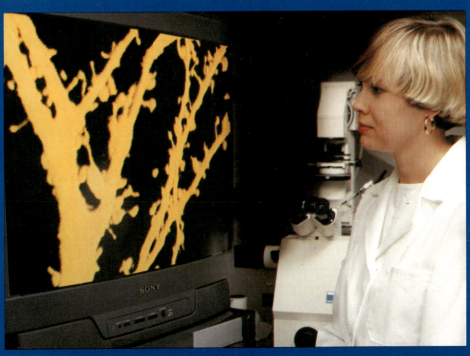

1990s

NASHVILLE MEDICINE
A History

JAMES SUMMERVILLE
Foreword by U.S. Senator William H. Frist, M.D.

Association Publishing Company
100 Oxmoor Road, Suite 110
Birmingham, Alabama 35209
(205) 941-4623

John Compton, Publisher

Published with cooperation and assistance of
    Nashville Academy of Medicine: David R. Yates, M.D., Chairman of the Board;
    John W. Lamb, M.D., President; Margaret Click, Executive Director

Book Design by **Lenore B. Corey / Brewer Design Company**

Dust Jacket Design by **Bonnie Henson / The Graphic Underground**

Photo credits: Tennessee State Library and Archives; Annette and Irwin Eskind Biomedical Library; Photographic Archives, Vanderbilt University; Meharry Medical College Archives; *Journal of the Tennessee Medical Association*; *Southern Practitioner*; *Nashville Journal of Medicine and Surgery*; W. W. Clayton, *History of Davidson County, Tennessee* (J.W. Lewis, 1880); Tennessee Christian Medical Center; Archives of St. Thomas Hospital; Baptist Hospital; Metropolitan Nashville General Hospital; *Art Work of Nashville* (The W. H. Parish Publishing Co., 1894); Tennessee Medical Association; Archives of the Metropolitan Government, Nashville and Davidson County; American Red Cross; U. S. Department of Veterans Affairs; The Frist Clinic; U. S. Senator Bill Frist; Tennessee Women in Medicine; Cumberland Science Museum; Nashville Academy of Medicine

Research associates David Logsdon and Tina J. Tope ably assisted the author with the gathering of photographs.

CONTENTS

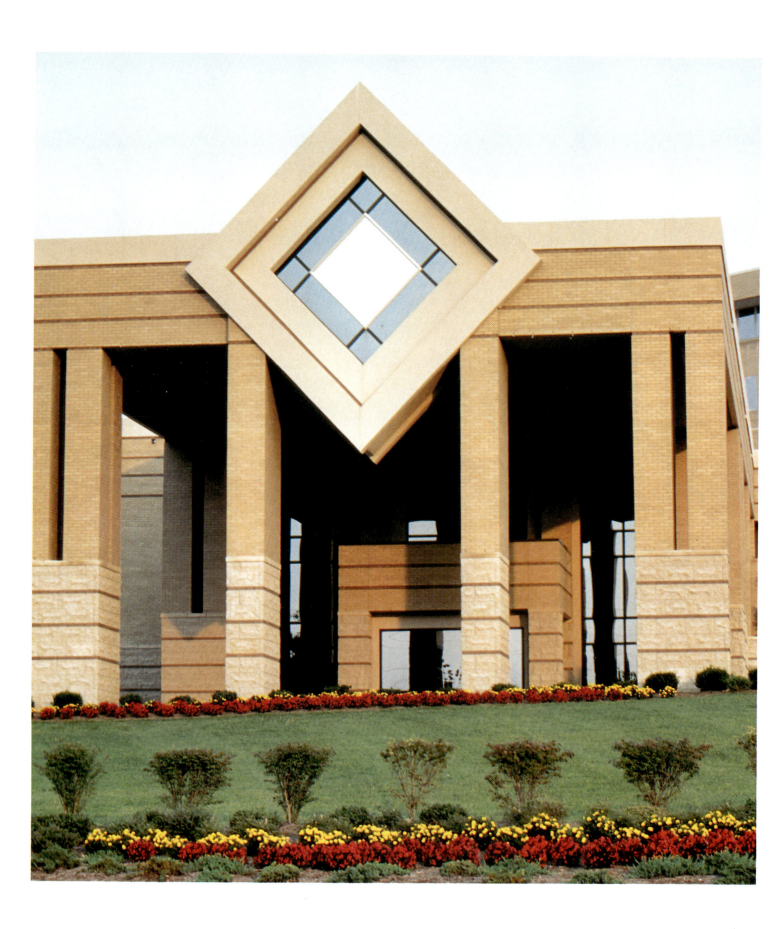

FOREWORD

few communities in America are as steeped in the tradition and practice of medicine as Middle Tennessee. With two prominent medical schools (one historically black), scores of innovative individual and group physician practices, numerous comprehensive private and investor-owned hospitals, a nationally-recognized science and research infrastructure, various creative and dynamic delivery systems, and more new start-up health care companies than any city in the nation, Nashville today is a rich amalgam of medical excellence and state-of-the-art care.

The roots of this story are artfully surveyed in the following pages by James Summerville, from Nashville's earliest days through wars, epidemics, political and social changes, and the synergies of collaboration within the medical profession. Weaving the lives of physicians with their times, Summerville traces the evolution of medical schools, hospitals, and organizations of doctors. The close bond between the history of our city and the medical profession recalls the vision of a former President of the Nashville Academy of Medicine, John C. Burch, who said in 1947: "All of us are committed to developing Nashville as a great medical center . . . . Our goal [is] Nashville, the Medical Center of the South."

The recent association of Meharry and Vanderbilt extends that vision; indeed Nashville is rapidly becoming the "health care capital" of the nation. And on the eve of a new millennium, we can, in the words of Dr. John W. Lamb, "do things previously impossible in the history of mankind."

By recording this story, James Summerville has made a wonderful contribution. Limited by space, this book is necessarily incomplete. The only frustration in reading it is to cry out for more! Yet, it will inspire future historians to preserve other details and capture other moments.

In my own life, I have been blessed to witness the more recent history of medicine in Nashville by growing up in a medical family, with a physician dad and two physician brothers — one a cardiac surgeon and the other a surgeon-turned hospital businessman.

With the eyes of a six-year-old, I admiringly watched my father depart every evening after dinner, black bag in hand, to tend to the needs of others. I observed Nashville medicine as a 10-year-old, making rounds with Dad at the old St. Thomas Hospital, and stealing a glimpse of those fearsome contraptions known as "iron lungs."

Then in the early 1960s, there was that first EKG machine — a technology mind-boggling at the time — hooked up to the telephone in Dad's bedroom so that in the middle of the night he could interpret the etiology of a patient's chest pain in some distant town. And at age 15, I recall vividly my family sitting around the dinner table at our home on Bowling Avenue when my oldest brother, Tommy, finally convinced Dad that basic business principles should apply to hospitals — thus witnessing the birth of what became the largest hospital management company in the world.

Years later, as a medical student at Vanderbilt, I spent a summer working in the cardiac physiology lab. When my brother Bobby, a heart surgeon, was attracted back to Nashville to practice, I knew that I, too, would pursue that specialty. When I completed my training, my home town offered the perfect environment for nurturing a heart and lung transplantation program with top-notch research opportunities.

Many Nashville physicians profiled in the following chapters worked to influence public policy. Likewise my Nashville medical experience lent impetus to my decision to serve for a time as a citizen legislator in the United States Senate, where I could focus on the health of a nation.

Nashville has a unique place in American medical history, and this volume deepens our perspective on it. For that, I am deeply grateful to the Nashville Academy of Medicine, James Summerville, and the individual physicians and their families who have generously shared in preserving this extraordinary story.

William H. Frist, M.D.
U. S. Senator, Tennessee
February 1999

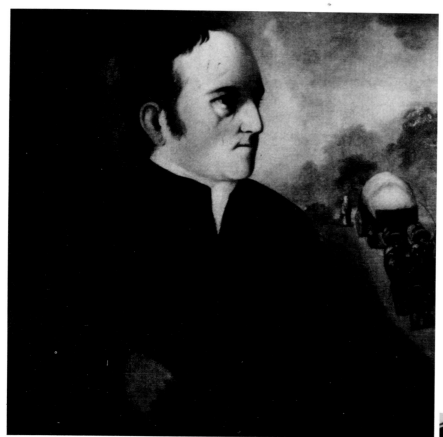

James Robertson, one of
the founders of Nashville

His son, Dr. Felix Robertson

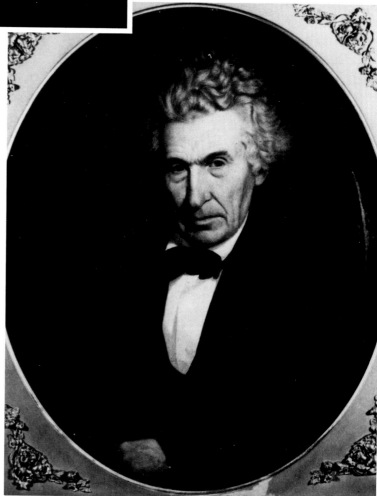

Chapter One

FROM ABORIGINAL TIMES TO FRONTIER TOWN

Through all the ages before the first human set foot in the Tennessee River valley and the Cumberland country, there flourished on its green hillsides a herbarium, a pharmacopoeia. In the fall there was the lowing of buffalo, in the spring the twitter of mockingbird, in the summer the splash of bass in the streams. And all the wild plants of the thickets and canebrakes and creek bottoms fed the creatures.

Several cultures of aboriginal people built settlements and cities on and near the place that would become Nashville. They kept nothing that we call history, and about them we know precious little, mostly based on archaeological investigation of gravesites and contacts recorded by the European explorers and the later settlers. Scholars tell us that some tribes recognized a priesthood of medicine men.

By the time settlers entered the place now called Tennessee, this priesthood taught the young hunting and other essential instruction, in courses that might last twenty summers. The most advanced teaching was in medicine-making. This medical training included a deep respect for the power of the spirit in a patient's health.

The Indians believed that illnesses were caused by malevolent spirits intruding on the body and that they could be cured with herbal remedies—providing the healer knew how to apply them against those spiritual forces. The healer administered the herbal medicine, then made a song or chant to call in a spiritual adversary of the spirit that had broken into the sick person's body. That enemy was sometimes assumed to have left a foreign object inside the victim, and the healer might by slight of hand extract the hurtful thing, then wave it above his head to show those gathered round. Many Cherokees also believed in the power of polished quartz and carried it as well as other amulets.

Individuals did their part to stay well. Southeastern Indians were careful to lie down to sleep with their heads away from the west, a source of bad spirits. Some averted the face of the mole, fearing it might pass along its weak eyesight. All meat for eating was well-cooked, as the sight of blood was taboo. The screech owl was believed to prophesy death, and the priests with medical training had formulae for keeping it away.

While they did not know the biology of infection, the aboriginal people living in the future Tennessee understood the importance of physical cleanliness. They bathed in the rivers or creeks, even in winter, and sometimes followed it with a sweating ritual. Like the administration of remedies, they believed that this icy plunge and heated bath cleansed the spirit as well as the body. We infer the last, because they exempted some people—women, the old, the sick. Anyone else who failed to take care of personal or household hygiene might be punished; the Chickasaws scratched them.

By the time settlement spread down the Appalachian chain and from North Carolina westward, the old Indian towns had been abandoned, but Chickasaw and Cherokee still foraged for game in present-day Middle Tennessee. These tribes could tell nothing of their predecessors, who had left the stone graves in today's Belmont neighborhood or the great mound near U.S. 70 just south of Bellevue.

Medicine men remained in high esteem for years after white conquest attenuated the natives' way of life. As they took up trade and made military alliances, their old ways gradually disappeared. For a long time, for sixty years at least after Nashville was founded, the Cherokees held onto their respect for their own priests and conjurers, who claimed to be able to thwart the epidemics of smallpox and consumption that plagued them. Even in the mid-1840s, the tribe's reputation commanded enough respect to sustain publication in Chattanooga of *The Cherokee Physician*; or *Indian Guide to Health*, which purported to offer "general rules for preserving health without the use of medicines."

MEDICINE ON THE NASHVILLE FRONTIER

Trudging over miles behind a horse in ill-fitted shoes, pioneer men and women often suffered corns and bunions, and the grease of bear meat helped a knife to sluice through and remove them. Rheumatism's inflammation cooled under a poultice soaked in rattlesnake's vital fluids, while wild onions squeezed and applied in cloth against a stiff neck might limber it. Draw water from an old stump, apply it against warts, and they disappeared, or so common knowledge had it. Even those low in body and spirit chanced improvement, if they drank a tea brewed from rabbit tobacco, also called "life everlasting." Remedies like these abounded in the dappled sunlight that fell under the Cumberland forests.

There was no body of generally accepted medical knowledge in those pioneer days. Every herb, every cure of any kind had its adherents and believers. Early Nashvillians came from a varied lot of Europeans, and each nationality held certitudes about drink, food, and ways of curing illness. If you ate a cucumber or a melon, some believed, you risked a fever. Drinking too much cold spring water could be harmful, advised Dr. Benjamin Rush, the nation's best-known physician. Some Cumberland country mothers gave their teething baby a dried meat skin to chew, while others accepted the truism that children ought not to eat meat.

Absent anyone with instruction in the medical arts of the day, "herb doctors" might be available to give advice, but generally each household had to provide cures for disease in both people and animals. Every household had its handwritten list of homemade remedies for all manner of illness. In a diary that he kept between 1790 to 1815, John Sevier recorded many remedies utilized by laymen in the care of illnesses and injuries. Cocklebur leaves boiled in new milk was pronounced "good for snakebite." Blue vitriol with half as much burnt alum ground into a powder would eat out a cancer wart, provided it was changed every six hours. Inflamed eyes would respond to chamomile boiled in new milk to a strong concoction, and so forth.

Men and women of the frontier were made strong by the conditions they lived under; hard physical labor required to clear a pasture or build a house and sleeping in cold rooms toughened a body. Still, cancers were common, and colds, influenza, and pneumonia made people miserable then as now. The most common diseases in early Nashville were rheumatism and malaria. Another dreaded scourge was smallpox. John Donelson's diary of the voyage of the *Adventure's* flotilla tells of a family that contracted the disease and was forced to travel at a remove from the main body of boats. Indians captured them, and their settlement was annihilated by spread of the infection. Historians of early times in Tennessee find little evidence of mental illness, addiction, or commonplace accidents.

FIRST SURGERY IN THE CITY

Caring for the sick was a duty that often devolved on the women, although James Robertson, one of Nashville's founders, seemed to have an intuitive gift for healing and performed the first surgical operation in the settlement.

On January 11, 1781, John Tucker, Joseph Hendricks, and David Hood left the Freeland's Station stockade to go to the bluffs, only to be fired upon by Indians, shooting from the canebrakes near the Sulphur Springs. Tucker and Hendricks were injured, while Hood was captured, scalped, and left for dead. When he did not return, a party from the fort set out from Fort Nashborough, and found him near death. They carried him back to the fort.

Robertson had returned that day from Kentucky where he had gone to acquire powder and lead for hunting and defense. He traveled to Freeland's station for the night and to see his wife who had just given birth to a son, Felix, the first male child born in Nashville. Next day, after helping fend off a nighttime attack by Chickasaws, Robertson returned to the bluff and went to see Hood. By the light of a grease lamp, he perforated the outer table of the skull using a shoemaker's awl. This allowed granulation tissue to grow up from the marrow and reepithelize the exposed bone. In about two years Hood had fully recovered, and lived a long life. Dr. Felix Robertson later recounted that his father had learned the procedure from a French surgeon traveling on the frontier. "We could therefore say," wrote Dr. John B. Thomison many years later, "that James Robertson was not only the founder of Nashville but the founder of Nashville medicine as well."

THE PIONEER PHYSICIAN

Some soldiers of the Indian and Revolutionary wars learned techniques for staunching blood or repairing wounds. On the basis of his battlefield experience, one "E. Winchester" doctored everything from asthma to trauma in the crude settlement on the bluff in its early days. Nothing is known of this man, but one may assume that he utilized the widespread methods of the day: bloodletting (although it was on the wane by 1800), and the use of powerful drugs more likely to kill than to cure, such as arsenic. Dr. Rush, an advanced thinker for his day, had some insight into the efficacy of prevention. He urged people to practice personal hygiene, get fresh daytime air, exercise, and practice temperance when it came to alcohol. One must note that the esteemed physician did not call for abstinence. The medical benefits of the toddy were widely believed in, and Dr. Rush, like most physicians of his time, sometimes prescribed a spirit, even for children.

A pioneer physician might possess a library that included treatises on surgery, obstetrics, anatomy, inflammatory illnesses, anatomy, fevers, purgatives, and various dictionaries, compilations of physicians' testimony, and animal illness. He carried forceps for pulling teeth, and small quantities of commonly used drugs, such as vitriol, opium, sugar of lead, and a dozen more. His saddlebag in addition held syringes, Spanish fly, and leeches. Surgical gear might include a hook, a gum-lancet, and a knife or two.

For several years "Granny Nell," an old Shawnee Indian woman acted as a "female doctor," while running a tavern on the square. Dr. James White, Middle Tennessee's first physician, arrived in 1784, five years after the Robertson party. He made his home at Hickman's Station, west of Nashville. Also a lawyer, he held numerous government jobs at one time or another. In 1786 there came Dr. John Sappington, remembered for his compounded pills covered with sugar coating, which were regarded as a sort of cure-all, working most likely as a

The Emergence of Modern Medicine

Frontier Nashville, remote from the scientific centers of Western Europe, did not know that medicine was undergoing great changes. As in astronomy and other physical science, medicine moved from an emphasis upon principles to an emphasis upon facts. Understanding the order of the universe came about not through logical thinking but through observation and experience—empiricism.

Researchers in Germany, France, and England were splitting medicine from its medieval traditions. When European monarchs incorporated learned societies to make scientific investigations, experimentation became fashionable. Under the influence of this experimental philosophy, physicians influenced by the attitude of the time must investigate, and think for themselves. What procedures actually proved most effective? Experimental and surgical pathology had their beginnings in the systematic and objective studies of John Hunter in London and his extraordinary collection of anatomical specimens. The measurement of blood pressure by Stephen Hales, muscular contraction by Albrecht von Haller, the basis for all future studies in the physiology of muscles and nerves.

Detailed observation in anatomy and physiology made possible the first systematic work in pathology. Clinicians acquired new facts and new viewpoints about disease, distinguishing between the merely abnormal and the pathological. The last half of the eighteenth century saw the first attempts at correlating clinical and post-mortem observations. A doctor at a bedside might note coughing and fever; another at dissecting table described the nodules in the lungs known as tubercles. The disease of consumption could be named only when physicians associated these phenomena. Now clinical and pathological findings could be compared. This way of understanding spread across Europe and America.

This intellectual climate was warming, just as James Robertson was saving the life of David Hood. English analytical philosophers like John Locke and David Hume were spreading the scientific point of view, the pursuit of knowledge through experience. One must reason, but about the data from the senses, rather than abstract notions, ideals, principles, absolute or transcendental things. The Enlightenment philosophies believed in a science of observation and of reasoning based strictly on it. Science became optimistic about results based in measurement and it became popular among educated people. Americans read of Franklin and his kite and elected as president Thomas Jefferson, the collector of fossils, architect, inventor.

Observation and investigation introduced into medicine procedures that worked. Digitalis has been an "old wives'" remedy, but study of patients showed its effectiveness, and it went into the books of *materia medica*. The common observation that fresh foods prevented scurvy became the basis for critical, empirical studies that proved the peculiar value of them, thus opening the branch of preventive medicine.

Abroad on both continents was a rising interest in public hygiene, such as the cleanliness of streets and water supplies and the abatement of nuisances associated with factories.

Edward Jenner's classic experiments, involving hypothesis and testing, led to vaccination, and protection against smallpox, the infectious bane of the Tennessee frontier. Vaccination was a mechanical improvement over inoculation, comparable to such tangible and useful contemporary accomplishments as the steam engine.

As Nashville was founded, Paris was becoming another world scientific capital, with brilliant and intensive work in mathematics, physics chemistry, and biology. In 1790s a number of able physicians began to apply empirical principles to medical studies, tracing clinical data to sources in organs with changes in latter analyzed to see the entire pathological picture.

Bichat's basic discoveries in the anatomy of tissues was another step toward a localized pathology, away from the old, general theories of humors or solids. By correlating bedside observations and subsequent pathological findings physicians arrived at distinctions between different disorders. The invention of the stethoscope proved of enormous value in diagnosis and encouraged examination, not mere observation, of patients.

Part of observation was correlation of records. In how many cases did the popular treatment of blood-letting result in the patient's improvement? In how many did it result in relapse, or worse? Record the statistics, and only then draw conclusions. Statistics demolished heroic methods. Exact studies showed that bleeding was of very uncertain value, and led to its discrediting.

French chemists found a number of valuable drugs during the first quarter of the nineteenth century. Morphine was isolated from opium, strychnine from nux vomica, and quinine from cinchona bark, The last was widely used in the frontier South and afforded some control of the serious malaria problem there. Studies of the various emetics and purgatives resulted in substitute of epsom and glauber salts for the much abused calomel. Bleeding and sweating had been good, supposedly, for every conceivable condition, while new drugs limited to particular purposes.

Still, much more would have to be learned about how the human body worked before scientists, then doctors, then people allowed for complexity. Hence the popularity in Nashville and elsewhere of the systems, characterized by monistic pathology and therapeutics. Benjamin Rush, best-known American physician of his day, argued in 1789 that all diseases could be reduced to one, and all treatments likewise. "The proximate cause of disease is irregular convulsive, or wrong action in the system affected." His students followed his prescription—heroic treatment, mainly blood-letting or purging that reduced convulsive action by depleting the patient, exhausting him. When Rush died in 1813, he was proclaimed the greatest physician the young country had produced. Yet the next generation renounced him.

When a doctor embraced a system, he was inclined to invest his whole self into it and promote it vigorously, while damning all others. Contention marked medicine in the West and in Nashville from the latter's founding until the profession organized early in the twentieth century. We may charitably assume that most doctors were intellectually honest, and believed that they comprehended the one way of understanding and curing human frailty. Every school claimed the experimental method, and insisted that the best results belonged to it.

Homeopathy was one of these. All diseases (except two) were viewed as forms of "the itch," and a single scheme of treatment recommended. Hahnemann's system appeared just in time to be subjected to exact and critical analysis, notably by French clinicians, who found its claims unsubstantiated, misleading, and unreliable. As a result homeopathy was forced out of regular medicine.

placebo. At an appointed time each morning, he stepped outside his office and rang a bell, proclaiming that it was time to take one of "Sappington's Pills." He was soon followed by his brother, Dr. Mark. The medical community swelled in number with Dr. Francis May's arrival in 1790. Then, adumbrating the professional conflicts to come, Dr. May became embroiled in argument with Dr. Frank Sappington, son of John, and killed him in a duel.

Whether these doctors added to anyone's store of years is questionable, but as in the case of the gunfight, they provided ample topics for public comment and conversation. Mark Sappington sported fancy clothes, including gleaming silver buckles that he wore at his knees and on his shoes. Generally regarded as a learned man, Dr. James White was apparently an alcoholic who would knock down anyone who refused to drink whisky with him. Dr. Hays, whose first name is not known, came to Nashville in 1801 and seems to have cut a figure for a time. He also fought a duel, but died, penniless, of delirium tremens.

The general repute of physicians of the day may be inferred from a provision in the constitution of the State of Franklin, formed in 1783-85 by political leaders in western North Carolina largely in the interest of securing their private fortunes in land. Its organic document excluded doctors, along with clergymen, lawyers, immoral men, Sabbath breakers, profane swearers, gamblers, and drunkards from holding public office. Some of Nashville's early doctors came, lingered, moved on; some were charlatans or with negligible training, but others possessed sterling credentials for the time.

AN ATTEMPT AT ORGANIZATION

The city grew south and west from the riverfront. By the late 1790s it was safe from Indian attacks. Soldiers of the Revolution or those to whom they sold, held vast tracts of land, where they felled trees cleared pastures and planted cotton, tobacco, and corn. In town a small mercantile and trading class began accumulating modest wealth. These conditions attracted physicians in great numbers, and they entered into vigorous competition with one another. Fees were high. If a doctor had to travel three miles, he presented a charge of three dollars, about what an unskilled laborer earned in six days. Once at the patient's bedside, more charges began mounting up for drugs, plasters, leeches, or hot toddies. Still, it was common for a Cumberland country doctor to have a long ledger sheet of accounts receivable or to take payment in potatoes, cured meat, or firewood.

Soon the supply of physicians exceeded the demand, naturally leading some practitioners to try to undercut their fellows in price. Other doctors sought to form an organization with all members pledging they would take fixed fees for prescribed services and never less. But medicine in Nashville and in early America was a small business; anyone could set himself up in practice and charge what the market would bear. Since everyone had home remedies, could buy any drug for sale anywhere, or obtain any proffered cure if he could afford the price, even the best-educated physicians had no authority over the practice of medicine. Despite the promises made in newspaper advertisements, they also had few reliable remedies against most disease and illness. The plan to form Nashville's first medical society failed.

To supplement their unsteady incomes, some doctors on the Nashville frontier opened apothecary shops, drugstores as they were later called. Dr. James Hennen's was the first, in 1794. It offered cures for everything the good doctor could diagnose, with jars and vials of ipecac, asafetida, myrrh, pomegranate root ground into powder, calomel, and an emulsion made from sawdust of a willow tree.

By about 1820 more than a dozen doctors were advertising in the local newspapers. A Dr. Dulany claimed to be able to treat sufferers from "cancers "of every description, wens and tumors, tetters, scald-heads, scurvy, scrofula, venereal diseases, gouts, rheumatism, sciatica, "and "troublesome and dangerous complaints" like consumption, female maladies, and blindness or deafness.

The best-known physician of Nashville in its first half-century was Dr. Felix Robertson, born on the night that his father repaired David Hood's torn scalp. Young Felix may have attended Davidson Academy, which his father helped found, but he began the study of medicine in the common way of the time, as an apprentice under Drs. Joseph Hays and Thomas Claiborne. What was not common was his next step, enrollment in a medical college, in fact the best one in the young nation, that of the University of Pennsylvania, whose leading light was the esteemed Benjamin Rush. Robertson took a diploma in 1806. His essay on "Chorea Sancti Viti" attempted to describe a nervous malady that attacked large numbers of persons on the frontier. The following year he set up practice in his home town.

Dr. Robertson deserves a biography of his own, and this short study can give only an outline. He helped found the Medical Society of Tennessee in 1830, the ancestor of today's Tennessee Medical Association, and served as its president. In 1827 he was elected mayor of Nashville. His business and civic activities included service as president of the Bank of Tennessee and trustee of Cumberland College and its successor, the University of Nashville.

A sign on Dr. Robertson's office wall read, "Never use medicine except when absolutely necessary." Apparently many of his colleagues trusted that precept. According to one of them, "Dr. Robertson has doctored more doctors than any doctor in Nashville."

He lived to see the Civil War. He opposed secession, but resented the North's invasion of the South and its capture of Nashville in 1862. He died in July, 1865, as a new world was being born. One of his patients who had had a broken bone set by Dr. Robertson lived to see the development of x-rays.

A contemporary and peer of Robertson, Boyd McNairy came to Nashville about 1790 from his native place in North Carolina. Two years before, an older brother, John, arrived with a party of settlers, among them Andrew Jackson. Boyd McNairy enrolled in Davidson Academy, where he finished in 1803, and that same year entered medical studies at Pennsylvania. He married Anne Marie Hodkinson, daughter of a wealthy shipbuilder, and the two of them returned to the little village by the Cumberland.

McNairy was a Federalist, and later as a Whig, opposed the politics of the Democrat's star, Andrew Jackson. He became a local champion of Jackson's great opponent, Kentucky senator Henry Clay.

Ironically, in the summer of 1813—the year before Jackson's astounding victory at New Orleans catapulted him into national fame—the General was wounded in a pistol fray on the market square by two brothers, Jesse and Thomas Hart Benton (the latter to become a highly influential U. S. Senator from Missouri). Dr. McNairy moved to his aid and had him carried to his office nearby. He saw to his care for ten days, before Jackson could go home to the Hermitage.

Still another alumnus of the great Pennsylvania school, Dr. John Shelby served with Jackson as a surgeon in the War of 1812. Wounded in the head, he lost sight in one eye, yet he returned home to amass considerable wealth through speculative land dealing and to found a college of medicine that bore his name.

In Europe of the Enlightenment, the modern world began, and science was driving the Industrial Revolution, even as the oars of flatboats plied the waters and wooden rudders turned John Donelson's flotilla into the Cumberland in the spring of 1780. Medicine was moving from an emphasis upon principles and systems to an emphasis upon facts. Understanding the order of the universe came about not through logical thinking but through observation and experience—empiricism. But there would be an epic struggle in Tennessee between empirical medicine and its challengers.

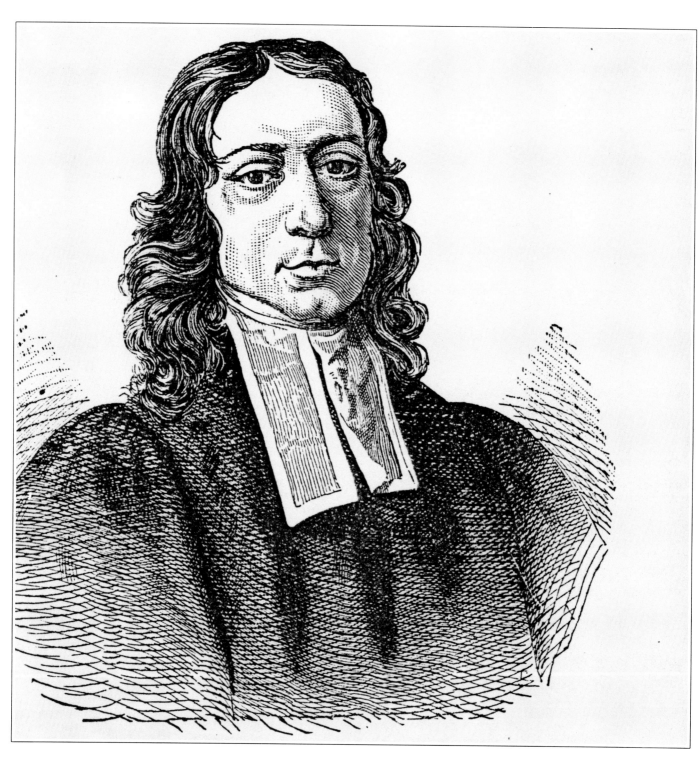

The Reverend John Wesley

Chapter Two

EMPIRICAL MEDICINE AND SECTARIAN CHALLENGE

*N*ashville's first church built on the public square in 1796 was raised by the Methodists, whose founder, John Wesley, taught that every man, and woman was perfectly competent to treat bodily ills. His *Primitive Physic* first appeared in 1747 and reached America in 1764.

John C. Gunn's *Domestic Medicine* went into dozens of printings and eventually claimed more than one hundred thousand copies sold. It promised the reader to describe "in plain language free from doctors' terms the diseases of men, women, and children, and the latest and most approved means used in their cure." Thus read the subtitle of the eighth edition, published in Pumpkintown, Tennessee by S. M. Johnston in 1839. It and its many imitators often emphasized diet and prevention of illness, advice and counsel given by many doctors.

Purveyors of patent medicine and homeopathists challenged medical school graduates. Perhaps the most popular challenger to empirical medicine in early Tennessee was the botanical system. Its founder, New England native Samuel Thomson, had no formal education when he set himself up in practice as a doctor. In 1809 one of his patients died, and he was tried for murder. When the jury returned a verdict of acquittal, he and his ideas about how to cure illness became famous. Four years later he patented his system of botanic medicine, giving him the legal right to sell what amounted to franchises in his methods. Thomsonian healers spread from his native heath into New York, then beyond. In Ohio, he claimed, half of the population rallied to his banner; his critics said it was only a third.

One of the appeals of Thomson's system was its simplicity. Cold

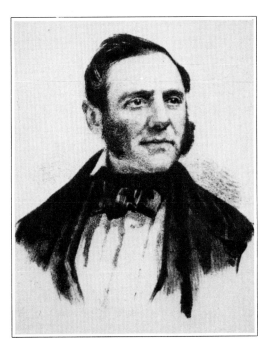

Dr. John C. Gunn

caused all disease, and heat was the remedy. All living things comprised the elements of earth, air, fire, and water. The solids comprised earth and water. Life and motion drew on air and fire, or heat. A diseased body could be restored to health by restoring heat, either through clearing the digestive tract so the sufferer could absorb food or indirectly, by causing perspiration. Thomson's basic prescriptions followed: a violent expurgative made from the herb *lobelia inflata*, red pepper, and steam baths. He specifically condemned any mineral remedy, favored by the medical profession.

By 1839 Thomson claimed to have sold 100,000 rights; Tennessee people bought some of them, and local presses turned out herbal healing books based on Thomson's system. *The Botanic Physician*, or *Family Medical Adviser* described more than 200 "vegetable remedies" and recipes for preparing and administering them. Its alleged author, A. H. Mathes, of Madisonville, Tennessee insisted that the system was "founded on correct physiological principles," and his 1837 book offered a "brief view of anatomy, physiology, pathology, [and] hygiene." One James M. Pearson offered still another treatise emphasizing herbs and roots as the cure for "all cases of disease for which the human family are subject," *The Sick Man's Companion; or Family Guide to Health* (Madisonville, 1836).

Even Adam G. Goodlett, one of the founders of the first Nashville association of doctors, lent his name to such a volume, *The Family Physician; or Every Man's Companion* (Nashville, 1838), which employed in the subtitle the democratic manifesto: "Every Man His Own Physician."

Homeopathists and Thomsonians won patients who doubted the claims of doctors promising other medicines and therapies. Indeed, many of their methods—leeching, bleeding, dosing with calomel, drastic surgery—were reviled and distrusted by many. Homeopathy's emphasis on infinite dilutions of harmless drugs provided a symbolic counterpoint to the "heroic" measures of even the most esteemed medical school graduates. By comparison, the "natural" therapies of the Thomsonians—emphasizing temperance, a healthy diet, and cleanliness—proved at least as effective.

These systems of medicine flourished in Andrew Jackson's home state and across America just as his political star was rising. In many ways the messages of both were the same. Health and healing were fundamentally not complex; anyone could study and learn what worked. Jacksonian Democracy called for the participation of every man—at least every white man—in voting and government.

As that fact suggests, these various systems of early nineteenth century Tennessee medicine should be understood, not as fraud or superstition but in the context of the times. Some politicians argued that physicians with formal learning exercised tyranny over common sense just as aristocrats had long suppressed the peoples' rule.

Botanists, homeopathists and the rest sincerely believed that knowledge of illness and disease was simple and accessible. Just as anybody could cook a meal to satisfy his hunger, so anyone could administer relief from pain and sickness, Thomson declared. The corollary was that doctors claiming truer methods practiced deceit and did so by attempting to mask their ignorance through abstruse language and keep their patients in ignorance.

EXPANDING COMPETITION

The number of physicians in Nashville grew rapidly, along with the city. American medical schools—ranging from the top tier like the University of Pennsylvania to mere proprietary ones, like the University of Nashville—were turning out hoards of graduates. The nation's supply of doctors with diplomas multiplied over 50 times from the first decade of the century to the 1850s. The total number of physicians, adding those trained in apprenticeships and other extra-academical arrangements, multiplied from a few thousand in 1800 to 40,000 by mid-century. In that same period, the nation's population grew less than five times. The effect in many places, including Nashville, was to increase competition within the ranks of

Antebellum Tennessee provided a fertile field for a medicine based in laboratory methods and empirical studies to take root. One scientific agriculturist was physician Francis Haynes Gordon, who introduced bluegrass into Tennessee and helped to found the Tennessee Agricultural Society in 1839.

Physician John H. Kain (1759-1831) of Knoxville wrote with distinction on Tennessee geology, prior to the establishment of a state-supported geological survey in the year of his death, 1831. George Bowen, M.D., professor of chemistry and natural history at the University of Nashville, published distinguished papers on the chemical analysis of minerals. Ferdinand Rugel, who apparently practiced medicine in East Tennessee in the mid-1840s, collected, assembled, and described one of the foremost collections of eastern north American flora.

Other antebellum Tennessee scientists carved a road through the wilderness. Gerard Troost, professor at the University of Nashville, was one of America's foremost mineralogists. A Troost protégé, Tolbert Fanning, founder of local schools, promoted an interest in geology among farmers and lay people through several agricultural periodicals that he edited. Engineers Albert Miller Lea and Stephen H. Long did essential altitude determinations, surveys, bridge design, and topographical studies, while Matthew Rhea is remembered for the first map of the state that incorporated field surveys. Others helped establish a scientific discipline, an institution, or a technical field in the state. The modernist project in medicine traveled from the European laboratories to Tennessee over the routes they opened.

Yet medicine was more astute in analysis than sensible in remedy; description exceeded prescription. Doctors had few effective therapies and the best in the Cumberland country knew it, and allowed for it.

Physicians who had no common ground—not in training, not in theory, not in integrity—had no place to take a stand, and taking a stand was of almighty importance to gain advantage in competition. The marketplace required a medicine that worked.

The Nashville Medical Society became a "school in which scholars teach each other," in the words of Sir William Osler. Given the open-ended character of medicine, the plain observations that physicians shared with each other—the plain descriptions printed in the *Nashville Journal of Medicine and Surgery*—helped all. Here was not dogma or judgment but observed fact, the same basis that science claimed. "What worked" was what Nashville physicians wanted to learn, as they listened to essays and papers read before their medical society.

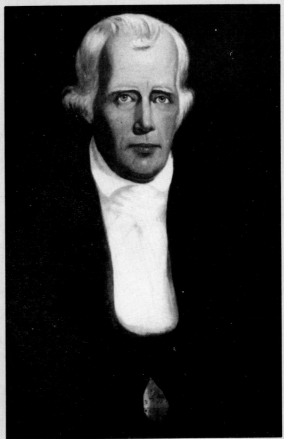

Dr. Gerard Troost

doctors. An historian of the city in the 1820s and 1830s notes the proliferation of their numbers, offices, and advertising.

No exact figures are available for the capital city, but an east Tennessee count, made by Dr. Frank A. Ramsey about 1850, found 201 physicians in a population of 164,000. Of these 35 had graduated from a medical school; 42 had attended one course of lectures but took no diploma; 95 professed to be doctors but had never received instruction except from reading a book; 25 were described as "botanics or steamers"; and two practiced homeopathy.

One observer noted that any farm boy too lazy to plow might procure a horse, a saddle bag, a lancet, a few dollars worth of drugs, and a copy of Gunn or Goodlett's book—and hang up a shingle as a doctor. Druggists also presented significant competition, and doctors responded to it. Some refused to treat any patient who used any proprietary or patent medicine against their advice. To meet the rising competition from apothecaries, Dr. William K. Bowling urged doctors to make and dispense their own medications. Well into the 20th century, many doctors did so, their office shelves lined with vials, stoppered jars, and corked bottles.

The misfortunate resident of old Nashville who summoned a doctor was liable to be bled by having leeches applied to his blood vessels; given an emetic to cause him to vomit violently; or a purgative that would send him repeatedly to the toilet. If these prescriptions did not cure him, or kill him, the doctor had others. Calomel caused the patient to salivate, and was given for various ills. Peruvian bark could be made into a foul-tasting concoction to stop chills. If the problem were a broken limb, there was a bandage—applied with the erroneous notion that it could not be too tight. For a toothache, the doctor carried an instrument that looked like a key with a hook attached, to twist the offending member out of the jawbone.

By contrast, physicians who had earned stellar reputa-

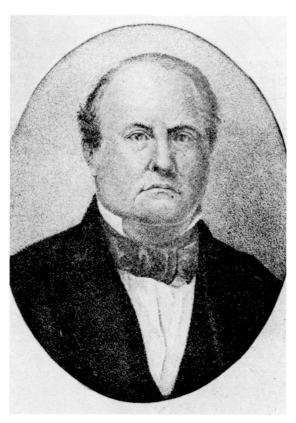

Dr. William K. Bowling

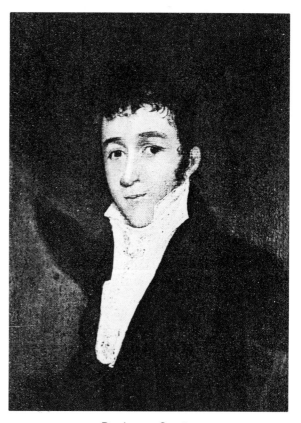

Dr. James Overton

tions among their colleagues worked in early Nashville. Dr. Adams Gibbs Goodlett studied with Dr. Benjamin Rush at Philadelphia, fought in the War of 1812, and won general respect in his practice in Nashville from 1817 to his retirement in 1848. Another Rush protégé, Dr. James Overton took up the practice of medicine here in 1819, living a long life until the late summer of 1865. He was remembered for his skill in removing bladder stones by surgery.

By 1814 Dr. James Roane had begun practicing medicine in Nashville. The son of Archibald Roane, second governor of Tennessee, he had taken a classics course at East Tennessee College (later, the University of Tennessee), and studied medicine in New York City. He was elected the first president of the Medical Society of Tennessee in 1830, forerunner of the Tennessee Medical Association.

In 1818 Dr. James Overton resigned his chair at the Transylvania Medical School in Lexington and relocated to the town on the Cumberland. He had been inspired and impressed by Dr. Ephriam McDowell's pioneering operation to remove a large ovarian cyst. An opportunity came for Dr. Overton to duplicate the feat but upon opening the woman's abdomen he detected that the tumor was mov-

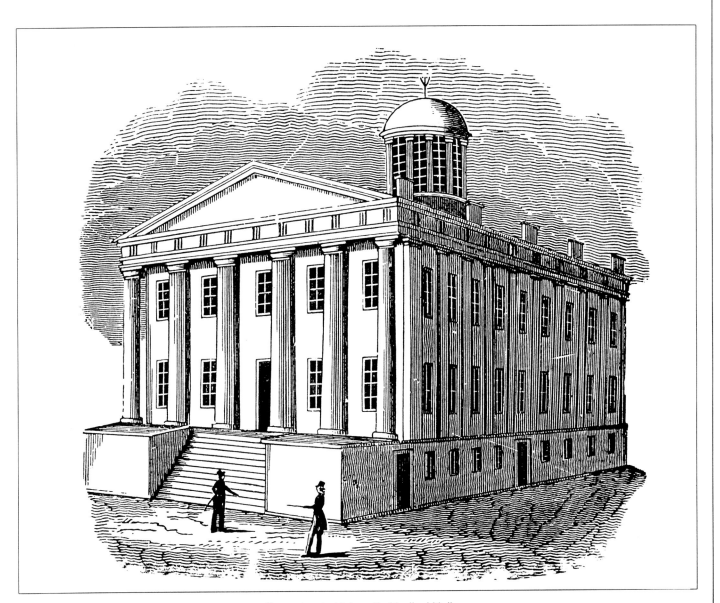

Transylvania University Medical Hall

ing. He closed the incision, and a few days later his patient delivered a healthy child. Although Dr. Overton confessed that his reputation suffered for a time, in 1821 he performed a remarkable operation for the time, removal of three stones from a sufferer's urinary bladder.

Dr. McDowell visited Tennessee in 1832 and performed the first successful ovariotomy here. In 1829 Dr. John Robertson Wilson described an abdominal operation for what he called "Ileus Attended with Intussusception," apparently the first instance of such a procedure. Still another Tennessee surgical first was a hip-joint disarticulation on a 14-year-old boy, done in 1859 by Dr. A. H. Buchanan. These and all surgical operations caused excruciating pain to the patient, since anesthesia was unknown until the 1850s, and probably did not reach Nashville until after the war.

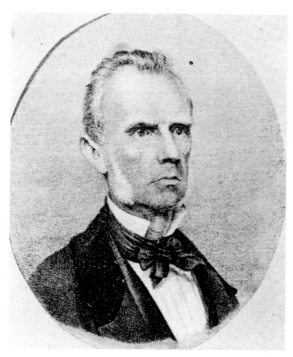

Dr. A. H. Buchanan

A SPLINTERED PROFESSION

Doctors sought respect and authority from the public, but experimental work being done in the laboratories of Europe were revealing that the medicines and techniques of even these highly educated physicians were nearly worthless. Prominent Nashville physicians openly expressed skepticism at heroic remedies like leeching.

By and large doctors of early Nashville, of early America, had no demonstrably superior treatments. Every practitioner could praise his own methods and damn those of his rivals. Many evidently did so. One scholar has observed, "relations among physicians in the early part of the [nineteenth] century can be described by one word— factiousness."

Eking out a living in a crowded field, lacking a medicine that worked, and facing a skeptical public, Nashville doctors turned to a time-honored method of besting the competition. They formed a guild, fixed fees for services, and excluded the practitioners of alternate systems.

In Boston, New York, and Philadelphia, well-educated physicians had also organized themselves into medical societies, and restricted membership to those who held degrees. Press and politicians deferred to the society when it came to questions of public health, and members often held appointments to the faculty of schools that their affluence helped to support. They treated people who could afford to pay their fees, and had no reason to cut prices.

The first organization of physicians in Nashville resembled these northeastern societies. It comprised elite doctors, and it sought mightily to regulate fees. The only surviving record of this society is a pricing schedule, dated March 5, 1821. Those signing "pledge[d] each to the other under the sanction of a solemn pledge and promise" not to charge less for listed services than the certain fees fixed for each.

Seven doctors took the pledge—Felix Robertson, James Roane, Boyd McNairy, A. G. Goodlett, and James Overton, whom we have met, as well as John Waters and R. A. Higginbotham. Robertson was listed as president of the unnamed group, Roane as secretary.

Four of these physicians—Robertson, McNairy, Goodlett, and Overton—had trained at the renowned medical school of the University of Pennsylvania. Roane had received a diploma from an unknown institution in New York City, while Waters was a graduate of the Baltimore Medical School, both probably proprietary institutions. He married a daughter of prominent Nashvillian and U.S. Senator Felix Grundy, which assured his social position. Of Higginbotham, nothing can be established.

McNairy had won a diploma; Goodlett had attended lectures; Overton, having previously studied law, learned medicine as a preceptor in the office of Dr. Benjamin Rush. McNairy became locally prominent in Whig politics, while Overton, evidently with the sponsorship of Henry Clay, served for a time on the faculty of the medical department of Transylvania University in Lexington, Kentucky.

Thus, the city's first medical society comprised highly-trained men who saw economic benefit and enhanced public esteem to be gained through association. The society drew such doctors and ignored (or was ignored by)

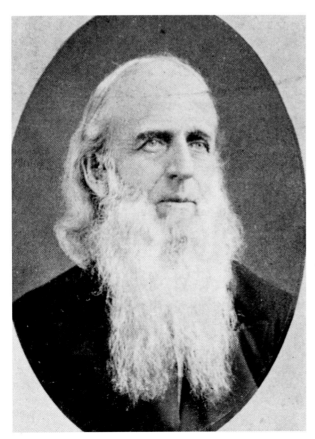
Dr. Charles K. Winston

the rest. It grew in membership, having 17 in attendance at the November, 1828 meeting. It took the name "Nashville Medical Society."

The question faced the Nashville Medical Society— should it become inclusive, and bring the homeopathists and Thomsonians under influence or control? Or should it insist on its members' qualifications and the small armada in their ken? Evidently, the group decided to remain an exclusive society. From the first, the privilege of belonging was limited to those recommended by their fellows as regular physicians. Consultation between society members and other kinds of practitioners was discouraged.

No homeopathist or Thomsonian or any other sectarian held office in the Nashville Medical Society. Dr. Charles K. Winston, elected president in 1844, belonged to the medical faculty of the University of Nashville. Dr. William K. Bowling, the president in 1853, had helped to start that institution. He personified the view that only physicians trained in medical schools were competent to treat sick people and to pass on the credentials of all who claimed they could do so. In 1851, the year he came from Kentucky to Nashville, Bowling founded the *Nashville Journal of Medicine and Surgery*, which he edited for the next quarter century. Bowling's journal called for a medicine that was one in dignity with law and theology, but free of influence from either. He opposed both state regulation of medical practice and endorsement of medicines by clergymen, a common practice.

CIVIC LEADERSHIP

Some of these same doctors distinguished themselves by taking part in the public life of the town. Institutions were few and small in antebellum Nashville. The city government, to pay for public outlays, resorted to private subscriptions, asking, for example, merchants on the Public Square to underwrite the cost of fire protection. When the call for a hospital was heard, in 1823, the General Assembly authorized a local lottery. Lending their names to the enterprise, if they were not actual sponsors, were Boyd

McNairy, James Overton, James Roane, and Felix Robertson. Here was the first hospital in Nashville dedicated to the benefit of people in poverty and the victims of mental illness.

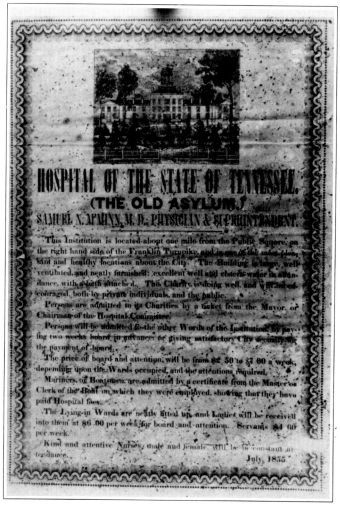

Hospital of the State of Tennessee: "the old asylum"

In 1832 a cholera epidemic struck the Mississippi Valley. Nothing was known about what caused the disease and how it was transmitted, but physicians suspected it to be a filth disease. Nashville was a foul place with open dumping of garbage, latrines that drained into creeks, and remains of slaughtered animals thrown into creeks, where they putrefied.

In mid-July the town aldermen created a permanent board of inspectors, charged with reporting nuisances, and directed that city employees clean the town of them. A committee on public health comprised Drs. Boyd McNairy, James Roane, Samuel Hogg, J. L Hadley, Felix Robertson, and James Overton. These physicians recommended strict measures: quarantine for persons suspected of communicable disease; purification of both public streets and private residences; and even prescribing diet, clothing, and hygiene for individuals.

In the winter and spring of 1832-33, the disease cut its swath, claiming among its victims Dr. James Roane. The sons and grandsons of these physicians would look the plague in the face again.

As Nashville grew from village to town, it divided along lines of economic and social class. In the days of the rude settlement by the Cumberland, all men and women were equal before the hard struggle of pioneer life. By the 1840s, some merchants had prospered, small fortunes had been made in cotton, investors in the new steamboat trade were turning profits. This commercial elite generally held the directorships of banks and served in public offices of a city government that had few powers and fewer fiscal resources. They welcomed into their midst those physicians who had distinguished themselves from the mass rank and file of doctors, in whom the public had no confidence. This distinction came about, not through effective therapies or even educational attainment, but social and family ties.

The University of Nashville's medical school vaulted some to this position, since a faculty appointment carried prestige. Others admitted to the town elite, drew on their connections: Adam Goodlett had studied with Rush; Overton had gotten help from Henry Clay to win a faculty appointment at Transylvania. It is not coincidental that the same names appear on the faculty roster, the public health committees—and the early medical societies.

Maturing an Organization

Yet the question remained, Who was a doctor? Was it anybody who made the claim and packed a saddlebag of medicines and a popular guide? Was it the physician who practiced a system, like Thomsonians, which explained all causes of disease in a common origin? Was it the doctor who apprenticed himself to another and rode the countryside delivering babies and treating wounds? Could an apothecary do as well by a sufferer as a doctor?

Most important of all: did a *bona fide* physician require a diploma? If so, what did that credential mean? How could patients—for that matter, fellow physicians—distinguish among the quality of education offered at issuing institutions?

A group of Nashville doctors sought to narrow these questions in June, 1853, when they formed the Davidson County Medical Society. Whoever was a "physician of good standing in his neighborhood among his professional brethren" could join. Yet the group determined to suppress those trafficking in systems, like the Thomsonians and the purveyors of patent medicines. Members pledged not to

> "advise or prescribe any of those nostrums, secret or proprietary medicines, generally called quack medicines, and which are hereby defined to embrace every compound preparation not recognized by the United State pharmacopoeia, and in which any one pretends to possess a private interest."

Members promised to cease attending patients who used such medicines against their advice, to buy any drugs they used only from apothecaries who did not dispense such medicines, and to boycott druggists who visited or prescribed for patients. Here was war upon competition.

Although the Davidson County Medical Society's first president, Dr. Wilson Yandell, held only an honorary M.D. degree, no less an orthodox physician than Dr. Paul F. Eve described him as the "leading practitioner of his section." William K. Bowling also delivered papers at its meetings.

What of the old Nashville Medical Society? Like most such entities throughout the nation, it apparently experienced periodic suspensions and reorganizations. Dr. Thomas Woodring, in a paper on pioneer medicine and early Nashville physicians, posits that the group "was functioning" during the hiatus in the historical record between 1830 and 1844. But Dr. Daniel Drake casts doubt on this view; on a visit to Nashville he found that the medical profession there was not organized into a city society but that it was the mainstay of the state association of physicians.

A similar gap occurred between 1853 and 1858, when no mention of a city medical society appeared in the *Nashville Journal of Medical and Surgery*. It is possible that such a city society lingered on, never being formally

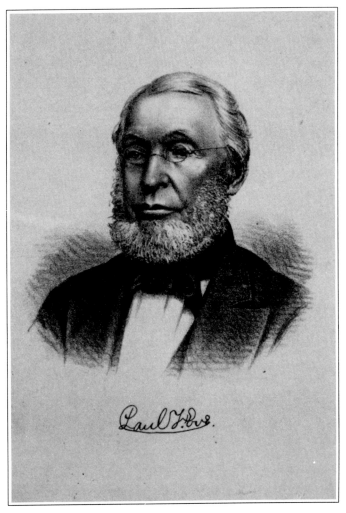

Dr. Paul F. Eve

William Walker, Physician and Filibusterer

Born in Nashville, William Walker, "the gray-eyed man of destiny," attended the University of Nashville and the University of Pennsylvania's school of medicine. He also held a law degree. With a passion for glory, office, and honors, the practice of his professions left him restless. He soon gathered a band of followers and began a career of private military action against other countries. When the Mexican government refused him permission to settle in *Baja* California, he invaded the peninsula with his band of forty-five men and on November 8, 1853, proclaimed himself president of new "Republic of Lower California." Mexico took exception to the violation of its sovereignty and dispatched troops, which chased Walker back across the border to United States soil.

Walker turned his attention to Central America, whose republics he regarded as client states of the United States and Britain, two great powers that rivaled each other for hegemony in the region. He decided to acquire one or more of them, planning to extend slavery there. In 1855 Walker appeared in Nicaragua, placed himself at the head of an established political party, and defeated his opponents. In May, 1856, the United States recognized his government, and a few months later he was inaugurated President of the Republic of Nicaragua.

El Presidente Walker returned to Nashville for a triumphal visit, his hometown citizens giving him a parade and a reception. He went on to Memphis where he was well received, too, many of his hearers promising money for his venture in Nicaragua.

These generous supporters did not realize that Walker's career had reached its zenith, and that he would be brought down by a powerful American businessman. When Walker took control in Nicaragua, he learned that Commodore Cornelius Vanderbilt's Accessory Transit Company held a monopoly on transportation and was amassing a fortune on the franchise, largely from ferrying fortune seekers bound for the California goldfields across the isthmus. President Walker promptly canceled Vanderbilt's concession and gave the business to a firm back in the United States, in which he and others who financed the filibustering campaigns held a large interest.

The Commodore retaliated by encouraging the President of Costa Rica to make war on the Nashvillian. Walker was driven out of Nicaragua in 1857. Twice he tried to regain power and twice was rebuffed. In his last attempt Walker made war on Honduras, which had joined his enemies in Nicaragua and Costa Rica. British troops received his surrender in 1860, promising not to turn him over to those enemies; almost immediately his captors broke their promise and handed Walker to the Hondurans. On September 16, Walker was executed by a firing squad.

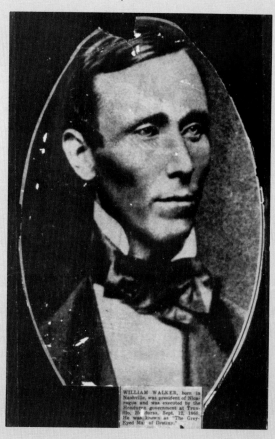

WILLIAM WALKER, born in Nashville, was president of Nicaragua and was executed by the Honduras government at Trux-Ho, Honduras, Sept. 12, 1860. He was known as "The Grey-Eyed Man of Destiny."

Dr. William Walker

dissolved but existing chiefly on paper. Sometimes a delegation from the University of Nashville's medical department represented the city's medical profession at the annual conventions of the American Medical Association, although the society was listed in 1854. When the AMA met in Nashville in 1857, delegations for both the Davidson County Medical Society and the Nashville Medical Society filed credentials.

When the Nashville Medical Society reorganized in June, 1858, Dr. A. H. Buchanan took the gavel as the first president under the new order. Like James Overton, he had attracted the support of Henry Clay for making a start in the West. After several unsettled years in eastern Tennessee and Louisiana, he began a preceptorship in medicine. Subsequently he enrolled at the medical department of the University of Pennsylvania. Two sessions of formal lectures were required for a diploma, but at the end of only one the impoverished young man persuaded a reluctant faculty to examine him and, upon passing, to award him the M.D. degree. At the University of Nashville he became professor of physiology and surgical and pathological anatomy.

Buchanan lamented the low prestige in the public mind of doctors trained in the same way as he. In the *Nashville Journal of Medicine and Surgery*, he wrote:

> "The physician of Science is put upon the same level and ranked in the same class with quacks. . . .There are at present no inducements, no rewards, no protection, no honors to help us in Tennessee to inspire and encourage the industrious and investigating student."

Raising public appreciation of the trained physician became a major object of the society under Dr. Buchanan's leadership. He called for, and the group adopted, a constitution that required all members to be "regular graduates in medicine from some respectable medical institution."

At the same time, the society moved to reinforce the economic well-being of its doctors. Members debated whether to adopt a "code of charges" drawn up by physi-

cians of the town "some years ago." Most were already party to the code, some insisted. Perhaps the original purpose of the 1821 medical society was carried on, even when a formal organization faltered or failed altogether.

It is not clear whether the reorganized society reaffirmed some sort of fee bill and bound members to it. But it did pursue another purpose, one that became increasingly important to doctors as they sought to make themselves into a profession. The new Nashville Medical Society established the office of health reporter to survey conditions of morbidity and mortality in the city. Dr. Charles K. Winston further proposed that physicians organized in the society solicit the city government to establish a board of health, sanitation laws then being solely in the hands of a weak constabulary. Before the town fathers could act, the nation split in two.

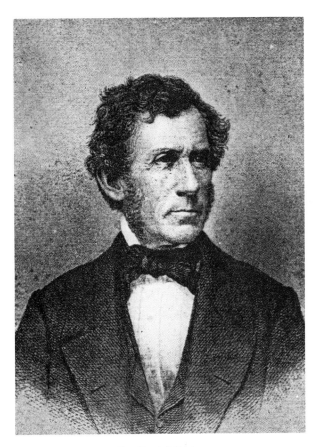

Dr. Daniel Drake

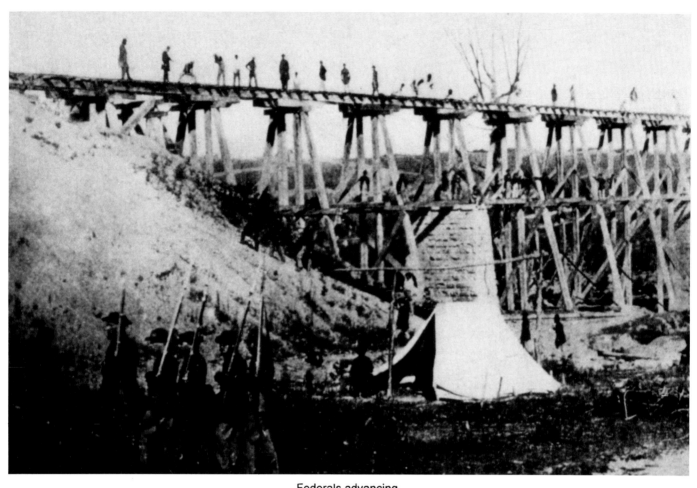

Federals advancing

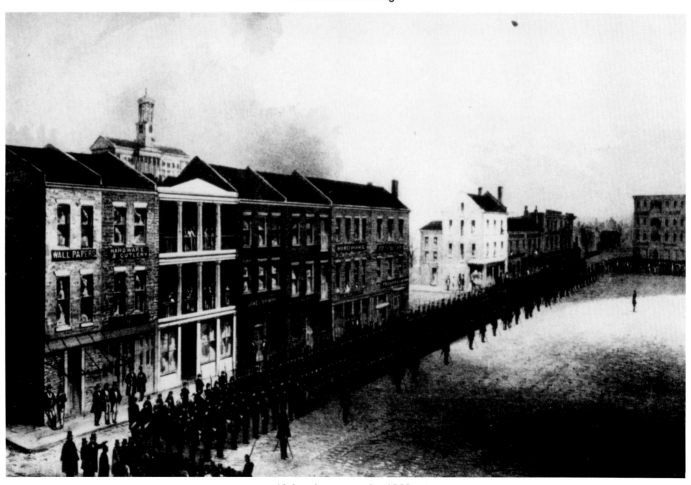

Union dress parade, 1862

Chapter Three

OCCUPIED CITY

---

*N*orth and South, everyone thought the war would last only a short while. The Confederacy went into the field without a single munitions factory on its soil, and underestimated the Union's technological capacity. The Yankee soldiers supposed their righteous brigades would smite the infidel, and then they heard the rebel yell, and the ferocity of rebel fighting boys fell on them.

Ulysses Grant's brilliant attack on Forts Henry and Donelson gave the North its first great prize, Nashville, after Confederate forces under Albert Sidney Johnston decided to withdraw. The city government might have set the town ablaze but chose peaceful surrender. General Nathan Bedford Forrest nonetheless supervised destruction of vast amounts of foodstuffs and armaments to keep them out of enemy hands.

From the day of its capture, in February, 1862, Nashville became a stronghold of Union forces in the western theater—an administrative, logistical, and supply center for the federal campaigns in the west. Naturally, it became a medical center as well. The city was served by rail lines and riverboats that could bring the wounded from the fronts in Tennessee, Alabama, and Georgia. After Shiloh in April, its conquerors knew what blood and terror lay ahead, and prepared to set up an extensive network of military hospitals and convalescent camps, impressing what they needed from private property owners.

The secessionists government of Tennessee had anticipated victory, but prepared for casualties. General Johnston, commanding the Confederate army in the west, handed the task of organizing a medical department to Dr. David W. Yandell. In the first autumn of the war, Dr. Yandell set up thirteen hospitals in Nashville. Troops took over homes and businesses when owners refused to rent them, filling parlors and hallways with cots.

To take charge of one of these hospitals, Dr. Yandell appointed Samuel Stout, a medical graduate of the University of Nashville and at the time a surgeon in the Third Tennessee Regiment. Dr. Stout's headquarters was Gordon Hospital, located in a warehouse on Front Street (later, First Avenue), opposite the wharf where cotton and country produce were loaded onto steamboats for shipment to Memphis or New Orleans.

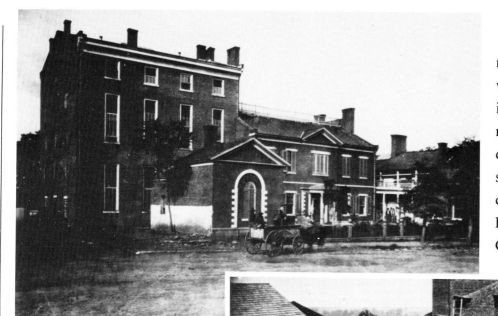

Stout toured the facility and noted its inadequacies. It lacked ventilation; its patients, numbering more than 200, had never been registered. He found himself in charge of a staff of three assistant surgeons, but in a facility without discipline, procedures, or order. Like most hospitals of its time, Gordon Hospital cared for either

A group of military hospitals

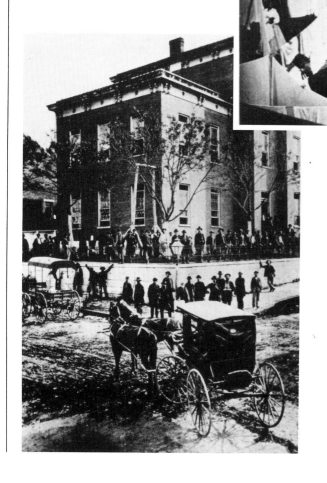

sick people with means who for one reason or another had no home or for transients who fell ill and had no place to stay. Soldiers of the war, of course, swelled this latter class as the savagery erupted on the battlefields. Surgeon Stout oversaw the cleaning and disinfecting of Gordon Hospital, and started patients on a dietary regimen that included fresh vegetables, butter, and eggs.

THE ARMY IN BLUE ARRIVES

Dr. Stout was enjoying his Sunday dinner at the City Hotel when a courier on horseback rode by and called out, "The Yankees are coming, are just below the city." He hurried back to his hospital and found his panic-stricken patients out in the street, some of them hobbling on crutches or shuffling, being too weak to walk. He sought to get them places on trains leaving town. But there was a massive exodus with every car filled and people even clinging to the roofs. Men who could walk from the hospital were ordered to a field south of town or to a convalescent camp.

The medical service also prepared to absorb the wounded from Fort Donelson. The confusion grew when a steamboat drew up at the wharf bearing Union prisoners needing medical attention. They shortly joined Confederate soldiers still under treatment at the Zollicoffer Barracks, and both were visited by volunteers from the Confederate Nurses Association.

Two hundred soldiers in pain or grievous hurt were gathered in an old granary. It had a muddy earthen floor, little medicine, no drugs to ease the suffering. Two stoves roared ablaze, but the air was damp. A visitor counted nine bodies, and thought twice that number of the living were in "death's last agony."

When word spread that General Johnston would surrender the city, the order that Dr. Stout had tried to institute at military hospitals began to fray as surgeons and assistants joined the general exodus. Some facilities were left filled to capacity.

Dr. Paul F. Eve was attending wounded Confederates at an overcrowded hospital, but departed abruptly to accompany to Augusta, Georgia, the remains of a private patient he had lost, a child, for burial in the family plot. When he tried to return to Nashville, Confederate authorities barred him, and he was posted as a surgeon at Atlanta.

John Berrien Lindsley, also a doctor and chancellor of the University of Nashville, took charge of the institution's hospital and it was clean, swept, and scrubbed.

He had expected and prepared for up to 300 casualties from Fort Donelson. They did not come, having found places in Clarksville to recuperate. But the Federal soldiers did, and surgeons from the United States forces quickly took over the buildings and grounds. On February 28, Dr. Lindsley surrendered his facility to a military surgeon on the staff of General Don Carlos Buell, who had taken command of Nashville.

Many of the sick and wounded now found new stamina and joined the migrant stream south, on foot, horseback, or railcar. But the Confederates were forced to abandon some sixteen hundred sick or wounded. The migration from the city continued for months, with families seeking refugee in the deep South behind Confederate lines. In the spring of 1863 Drs. A. H. Buchanan and John M. Watson joined the throng, as did medical colleagues John Henry Currey and J. P. Ford, a member of the medical faculty of the University of Nashville who been imprisoned on the charge of treason. Seven physicians had pledged to Lindsley that they would remain at all costs. These were Drs. William Bowling, William T. Briggs, Thomas Maddin, J. Dudley Winston, Charles K. Winston, A. A. Hatcher, and S. L. Wharton.

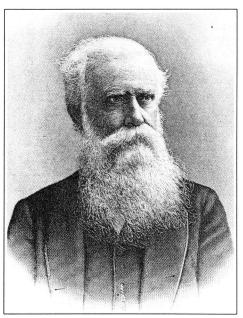

Dr. Thomas L. Maddin

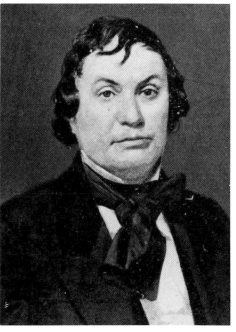

Dr. John M. Watson

COPING WITH CALAMITY

By mid-March the convalescent population swelled to four thousand soldiers, coping in hospital conditions that were uniformly terrible. Dr. Lindsley lacked enough doctors to cope. Fortunately, Union physicians arrived in numbers and with desperately needed supplies. For some time, Confederate and Union doctors worked side by side to perform surgery, dress wounds, and try to abate fevers.

That spring of 1862 the Union authorities opened twelve general hospitals and two regimental hospitals. Most of the places that had served the Confederacy just a few weeks earlier were abandoned. Seven of the new facilities were clustered around Rutledge Hill, sometimes called College Hill. There stood the home of the pioneer Rutledge family, and the University of Nashville.

These hospitals took in hundreds, at times, thousands of sick and wounded. The censuses fluctuated depending on the military action south and east of the city, the rate of discharge, or the return to home of ailing and permanently disabled soldiers. Sickness took more troops out of the fight than did minie balls or artillery fire. Yet the battlefield casualties told two terrible medical stories: no war as ferocious as this had ever been fought before, and its end was not in sight.

The Battle of Stones River began on December 31, 1862, and for the next three days Southern boys, under General Braxton Bragg, and northern boys, commanded by General William Rosecrans, charged each other, throwing themselves into withering fire, recouping and advancing again. The toll was terrible—Yank and Reb between them suffered twenty four thousand killed, wounded, or missing.

Nashville's hospitals were soon awash in blood, as ambulances and railcars brought the wounded to town. The Union authorities seized still more space, including the First Presbyterian Church, McKendree Methodist Church, and the First Baptist Church. At First Presbyterian the pews were ripped out, and more than a thousand cots put in their place. Several business houses were likewise turned into wards; even the Capitol became a harbor for the casualties for a short time.

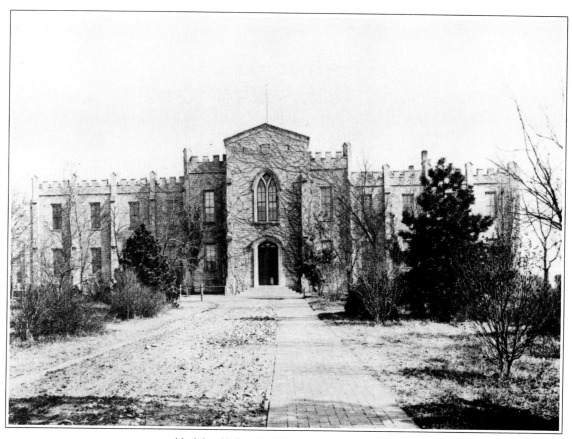

Lindsley Hall at the University of Nashville

It was still not enough, and some of the soldiers were sent to outlying towns. Gallatin absorbed three thousand patients, lying abed in more than thirty buildings. A local newspaper reported that Rutherford County was "one vast hospital" with Union soldiers resting and recuperating in every farmhouse.

As word of the massive slaughter sped north, the governors of Indiana, Ohio, and Pennsylvania dispatched physicians, nurses, supplies—and steamboats to transport the boys home. These hospital ships removed thousands, but the remaining population of "suffering humanity," said Dr. R. N. Barr, consumed energy and substance from the Union forces occupying Nashville.

Newspapers printed lists of casualties from both armies; by late January forty to fifty of the wounded died each day. Still the wagons lined the road between Murfreesboro and Nashville. On February 1, a number of Confederate soldiers were brought in, and some women of the city braved cold, rain, and mud to attend them. Brigadier General Robert B. Mitchell decided to punish their patriotism by giving them more of the same duty. He chose forty five wounded men and ordered them taken by stretchers to homes of three families who had supported secession. One of these was Dr. A. H. Buchanan. These assignments of Confederate wounded continued, doing little to relieve the overcrowded hospitals, but ground down some Southerners' pride under the Union bootheel.

By mid-year twenty five hospitals operated in Nashville. Dr. Ebenezer Swift oversaw this sizable apparatus, assisted by medical inspector George H. Lyman and staff surgeon A. Henry Thurston. Each hospital had a surgeon in charge and a staff whose numbers depended on the facility's size. Among these might be a master of wards, a steward, an apothecary, clerks, nurses, chaplains, and servants.

As the numbers of wounded from Stones River dwindled—due to death, departure, or recuperation—order returned. Dr. Swift and his associates paid attention to preventing disease, and received help from Army engineers to modify some of the buildings to introduce adequate ventilation. Aware of the need for balanced diets, the doctors gladly accepted help from members of the U. S. Sanitary Commission who rode the countryside and seized fresh vegetables from gardens and farms.

THE CHARNEL HOUSE OF NASHVILLE

General Rosecrans returned to Nashville on July 15, after an absence of several weeks helping with the pursuit of General Bragg. Next day he inspected the convalescent camps and the hospitals, among other fortifications and defenses of the great war machine that the city had become. (Accompanying him on this tour were two future Presidents of the United States, Military Governor Andrew Johnson and Adjutant General James Garfield.) Rosecrans soon returned to the front, in time to lead his forces against Bragg in the Battle of Chickamauga on September 19-20. In the forty-eight hours of the fight, more than thirty seven thousand soldiers were killed, wounded, or missing in action. Nashville families lost grievous numbers of husbands and sons.

Often missing an arm or leg or both, the luckier ones began arriving by railroad on September 24. An enlisted man from the 124th Regiment Ohio Volunteer Infantry, James Walsh from Cleveland, wrote in his diary, "We are well cared for here. I had my wound dressed for the first time in four days." One of his caregivers was a young nurse named Ellen Walsh of McEwen, Tennessee. Perhaps they talked pleasantly about sharing the same last name.

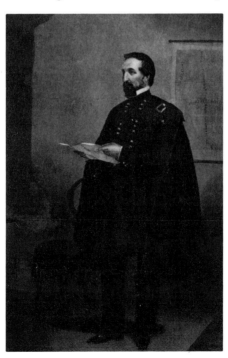

General William S. Rosecrans

Evidently they found more in common, as they courted, married, and settled in Nashville after the war.

Altogether five thousand sick or wounded men from Chickamauga poured into the city. Once again the governors of northern states sent physicians, and volunteers from charitable and eleemosynary groups—notably ladies' aid societies and religious orders—went from cot to cot in the teeming wards, swabbing wounds and changing bandages or whispering words of comfort.

Not all the suffering came from battle wounds. By 1863 venereal disease raged in the city, and Union authorities issued orders requiring prostitutes to undergo regular medical examinations. (This was possibly the earliest regulation in the United States of "the oldest profession.") Despite the premium on space, one hospital was assigned to treat women afflicted with these maladies and another was set aside for diseased soldiers. Both facilities became overcrowded. Love for sale had brought an epidemic to occupied Nashville.

Heroic medicine recommended harsh prescriptives for syphilis, gonorrhea, and the rest. Soldiers rebelled against them, and sometimes turned to local doctors. Dr. John White, a black physician and a botanic, won praise from an afflicted army sergeant, who praised him in a letter to Governor Johnson.

Despite the numbers of men it took out of the fight, prostitution continued to be practiced openly, and the Union commanders simply looked the other way. By September 1864, four hundred and sixty ladies of the evening were licensed to practice. In exchange they were required to submit to periodic medical examinations and, if found afflicted, to be treated at a special hospital. Some historians have called this the first attempt to control venereal disease through legalized prostitution.

Local physicians continued to see private patients, but practice in the occupied city held its dangers. The policy of Governor Johnson was to intimidate Southern sympathizers by arresting and imprisoning anyone who made any overt sign of support for the enemy. So instructed soldiers sometimes carried the order to the extreme and committed acts of violence against civilians. Dr. William Bass was leaving the William G. Harding residence (later known as Belle Meade Plantation) when two Union soldiers shouted for him to halt. He did not respond, and died from their shots. Although some press reports held that the doctor had been involved in a plot with some Confederate guerrillas, the killing was widely believed without justification and aroused great public antipathy toward Union soldiers.

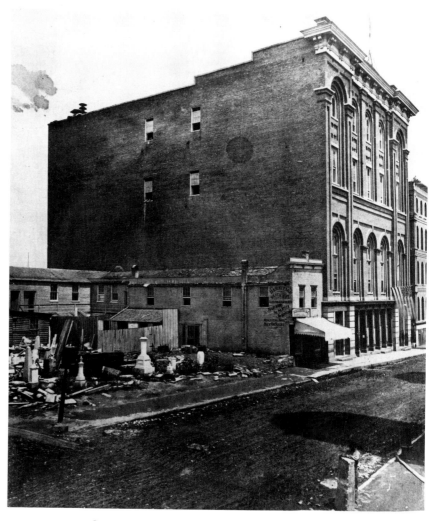

General Hospital No. 8 (the Masonic Hall)

Samuel Stout and Nashville's Civil War Hospitals

When Dr. Samuel Stout walked the premises of Gordon Hospital, and found an institution in disarray, he promptly drew up a strict set of regulations and ordered them enforced: a patient register was established; no one could leave the facility without permission; and visitors must register. He followed these with a still more detailed set of rules.

His sense of urgency can be understood when one looks at hospitals in the early nineteenth century. Rare in the South, these institutions in the northeastern cities cared for poor people without homes, or no one to care for them there, and people who were stricken while traveling.

Care of the sick was mainly done at home for the overwhelming number of people stricken with illness or injury. Thus, few soldiers had ever been inside a hospital. Wounded or ill, they had no choice but to repair to one since they could not go home. Despite the necessity, many objected. Doctors attached to the army's medical services were not much respected, nor did troops understand the need for sanitary care of traumatic injury or even personal hygiene.

Their physicians' knowledge may hardly have been more sophisticated. Patriots among doctors enlisted in the Southern cause that spring of April, 1861, but only the very few with military experience dealt with injury or pain *en masse*. Thus at Nashville's Gordon Hospital, Dr. Stout set out to manage doctors as well as patients, the former so they could cope with the overwhelming numbers, the latter so they could return to duty if possible.

Dr. Stout's great innovation was the movable hospital. When a post had to be evacuated due to enemy advance, he showed how their organization could be preserved, and bedding, medicine. and doctors travel on to a new location. By this competence, Dr. Stout rose to the top post in hospital administration in the Army of Tennessee.

In that position, he sought to have Dr. Paul Eve removed from administration of an Atlanta hospital on grounds of lack of management ability. Inspecting the facility, Dr. Stout had found filth, sputa, urine, and excreta on floors. Worthy of his lasting reputation among medical historians, Eve was coping with extremely difficult conditions; but Stout's concern was with the reputation of hospitals under his command. As he had done at Gordon, he closed, cleansed, and only then reopened his Nashville colleague's post.

The army Dr. Stout served was destroyed in the Battle of Nashville, and four months later the war ended. Dr. Stout never found a place in postwar America. He taught medicine at the Atlanta Medical College for a time, came back to Tennessee to farm, then returned to Atlanta to try the private practice of medicine. In 1874 he moved to Roswell, Georgia, and became interested in the afflictions of women factory workers, about which he published several papers. Neither prosperity nor professional success came his way, and he lived a peripatetic life as a public school teacher and part-time physician in his adopted home of Texas. In 1900, honored by his fellow physicians for a half-century in practice, he helped to found the Baylor University College of Medicine.

Through all those years until his death in 1903, Samuel Stout saved and preserved 1,500 pounds of hospital records from his service in the Confederate medical service. He had tried unsuccessfully over the years to find a job that would pay him a wage for writing a medical history of the Army of Tennessee. His archives passed to his children, who sold most of them to the University of Texas and other institutions.

DECISIVE BATTLE

For four long years of war, the history of medicine in Nashville followed the carnage on the battlefield. Morgan and Forrest would harass the enemy within the gates, lady spies would spirit intelligence across lines, but only in the great final battle for the city, would all be settled, the destruction of the Army of Tennessee, the end of Southern hopes for independence, and the fate of the United States.

At 3:30 a.m. on Thursday, December 15, 1864, bugles awoke sleeping Union soldiers and they stumbled through their camps in a thick fog. The artillery began bombardment, and fifty five thousand men took their places in the line that would lead the attack against the forces of General Hood. He possessed less than half as many men, and his line was stretched thin south of the city from the rail line running south of the city (roughly paralleling today's Fourth Avenue, South to Hillsboro Pike.) Far greater in numbers, the Union troops possessed repeating rifles, a technological advantage over the Southerners.

As the fog lifted, seven thousand soldiers under General James B. Steedman flung themselves across Murfreesboro Pike against the Confederate right. It fell back, but the main Southern line held fast. Although Steedman's forces were soon compelled to retreat to their original line, they did their job, which was to create a diversion. Hood watched carefully, but he had anticipated that the main attack would come on his left. About 10 a.m., it began, moving against him with men equal in number to his entire army.

Following the soldiers came volunteers with the charitable and missionary societies whose members had done duty among convalescents in Nashville hospitals throughout the war. They walked now in the direction of the coming danger.

By noon the massive Union right had crossed Charlotte and Harding Pikes and was poised just west of the five Confederate defensive positions, called redoubts, arrayed along Hillsboro Pike between present-day Woodmont Boulevard and Harding Place. Now the Union center,

under General Thomas J. Wood with headquarters at Belmont, could be ordered forward. Thirteen thousand were soon upon the Confederates. On their left, there came down the iron fist. Despite their brave and fierce resistance, by nightfall all five redoubts had been overrun and occupied by the Yankees.

Only darkness stopped the disaster. Hood's men prepared to make a stand again the next day. All through the night, the racket of shovels and spades could be heard, as the rebels dug trenches to make a new defense line in the Overton Hills, crossing the Franklin and Granny White Pikes. Meanwhile, by telegram, word reached President Lincoln of the Union force's first day's success. He replied, "Please, accept for yourself, officers, and men the nation's thanks....You made a magnificent beginning. A grand summation is within your reach...."

On Friday morning the Union ranks smashed hard against Hood's right at Franklin Road. They met withering fire from the low hills around the Overton plantation (Travellers Rest), but Yankee artillery replied in kind. One soldier was awed by the accuracy of the shelling, and noted that the creeks ran red with blood of killed and wounded men and horses.

That afternoon a unit of Union calvary swept around the Confederate left and gained the rear of its lines on Granny White Pike. At the same time the Yankees attacked with renewed force in the center and on the right, at Franklin Pike. "The hills shook, the earth trembled, the whole field was like the gaping mouth of hell," one eyewitness reported. At Shy's Hill, overlooking today's Harding Place, the rebels halted and refused to give way whatever the punishment.

About four o'clock Union troops began a general assault. East of Hillsboro Pike, troops from Minnesota led the charge across a muddy field, taking fire from muskets and cannon, but pressing on. Cavalry behind them, and with no hope of reinforcements, the Southerner's line collapsed. Shy's Hill was the last stand, and its brave defenders surrendered or fled south along Hillsboro and

Granny White pikes and the Franklin Road. The fight was over and with it all hope that the Army of Tennessee might relieve the beleaguered General Lee in the east. Four months later the Civil War came to an end.

On Saturday ambulances and wagons drove slowly over the fields, gathering the wounded and the dead. Now the Union commander took all the houses of worship in the city, without exception, for hospitals, and the court-rooms in the courthouse as well. Two thousand wounded, Southern boys and Northern boys, needed care as a result of the two-day fight. They were joined in a few days by the three thousand eight hundred casualties on both sides from the Battle of Franklin, which had taken place in November. Some convalescents were able to travel on, but more than seven thousand eight hundred remained in late December. By the time General Lee turned over his sword to General Grant at Appomatox Courthouse in April, the Union post commanders were relinquishing impressed properties. Nonetheless it held public school buildings and kept them in use as hospitals until late summer of 1865. For the last of the departed, the memory of the Battle of Nashville remained seared in their memory. As one witness wrote, it had been

"...a medley of soldiers disappearing in smoke, galloping horsemen, fluttering enigmas, rider-less horses, the prostrate dead and dying, trees splintered, cloudy hilltops. . .the roar of artil-lery, the sulphurous smell of battle smoke, the confused clamor of voices, the cries of the wounded and dying...an atmosphere overladen with death."

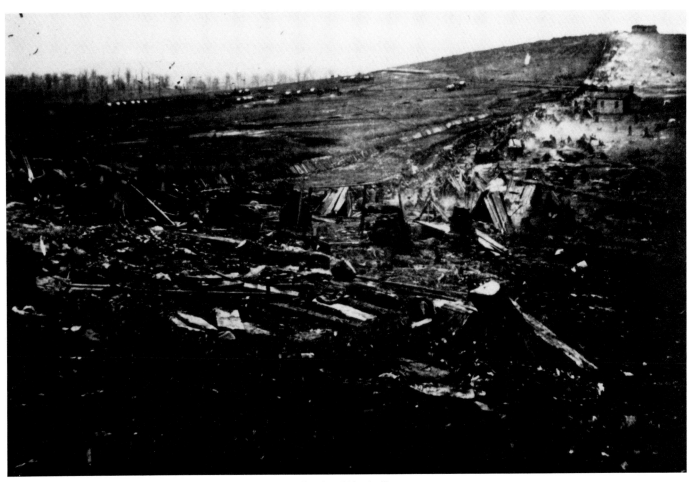

Battle of Nashville

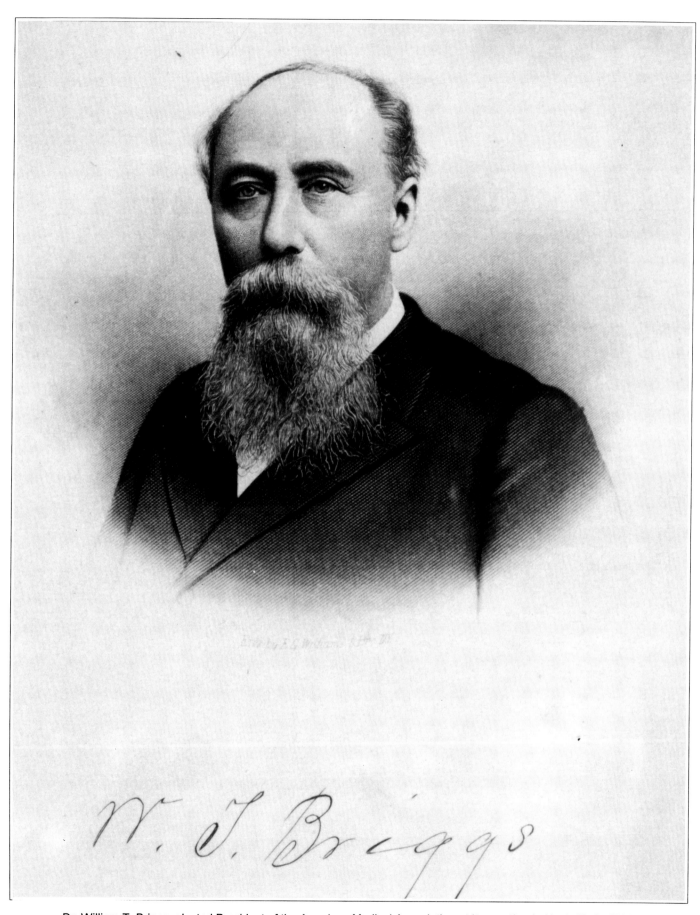

Dr. William T. Briggs, elected President of the American Medical Association at its meeting in Nashville in 1890

Chapter Four

BEGINNINGS OF THE NASHVILLE ACADEMY OF MEDICINE

———————————

$\mathcal{A}$fter a four-year hiatus, the Nashville Medical Society convened on August 16, 1865. Dr. Charles K. Winston, acting as president pro tempore, took the gavel as those present readopted the constitution that existed and resolved that no corporate or legal interruption had occurred. Forty one members were continued on the rolls, Dr. William K. Bowling, the senior among them in point of membership.

The following summer, when reports of Asiatic cholera created general alarm, the society urged the mayor and council to undertake public sanitation measures and to establish a board of health to oversee such work. On June 5, the society set up a board itself, naming two physicians in each ward and designating committees on hygiene, nuisances, endemic diseases, epidemic diseases, meteorology, and mortuary reports. Three weeks later the city council formally established the society's board as the Board of Health for the City of Nashville. Despite its attention to duty, cholera overwhelmed the city between mid-September and mid-October. Eight hundred Nashvillians perished in the plague.

The medical society regarded the pestilence as punishment to Nashville for long neglect of public sanitation. When city government passed into the hands of a Radical Reconstruction administration in 1867, the society and the health board endured more frustration. Mayor Augustus E. Alden refused to accept its nominee to head the health board. When the city was put into receivership by the courts, Alden's successor, John M. Bass trimmed the outlays for sanitary work.

It took another epidemic, in 1873, to establish the Board of Health on a permanent basis, with the cooperation of Republican mayor Thomas Kercheval. On the medical society's behalf, Dr. Winston claimed due credit for this success, adding that the society "thus established sovereignty over public hygiene."

Thus the way was laid open. The doctors represented in the Nashville Medical Society took the well-being of the general population in their care, and won their claim to represent the only true medicine. Not all these doctors yet accepted the germ theory of infectious disease—but the general suspicion of a connection between filth and epidemics was well-founded.

"THE FIRST NECESSITY OF REFORM"

On the eve of Nashville's centenary, the Board of Health took as its principal concern the abatement of nuisances, the inadequacy of the sewerage system, and the need for a pure water supply. Besides sharing certain members and officers, the Board of Health and the medical societies believed that public education concerning workable methods of preventive was the duty of both organizations. In his annual report for 1878, Dr. John Berrien Lindsley, City Health Officer, wrote: "The first necessity of reform is the enlightenment of the public mind. Sanitary science becomes a most valuable means of public education."

While ingratiating itself with the public through its concern with these civic matters, the Nashville Medical Society in the postwar years continued to serve the interest of members. In January, 1866, it adopted a fee bill, the list of charges having apparently been drawn up earlier and circulated among doctors.

Reports of "what worked" in particular cases of suffering provided the program at meetings. On September 6, 1865, the subject was the origins and etiology of diphtheria. Dr. John Callender insisted that the asphyxiating membrane could be broken up with the finger, and he recommended alcoholic stimulants as a remedy for the disease. Dr. William Briggs advised a tracheotomy when the larynx was occluded and related cases illustrating his opinion. When it came to trauma, gunshot wounds were commonly discussed, as were the results of accidents related to farm work. These last suggest how close the city and countryside still were.

Despite this practical agenda aimed at doctors and the public alike, within three years after its postwar revival the Nashville Medical Society once again faded from the historical record. Achieving and maintaining a membership of active participants apparently proved impossible. Certain unresolved tensions in the society's purposes may have contributed to the difficulty. If the group hoped to bring together all reputable physicians, then the measure of success was a long roster of members. But if the aim was to police the profession, the society had to become exclusive.

A still more fundamental problem lay in the flexibility of the medicine that most doctors of the time practiced. There was little therapeutic accord, and medicine's few effective methods were just as much the property of physicians trained in the leading medical colleges and the for-profit proprietary schools. At the same time, the economic self-interest of any given group of physicians dictated that the competition had to be limited.

The nature and quality of the education necessary to become a physician was the single most important issue facing American medicine in the late nineteenth century. The number of commercial medical schools continued to grow and with them the number of doctors. Between 1880 and 1900 approximately 60 new schools opened, an increase of over 60% in the total number. In this same period the number of medical students more than doubled. From 1870 to 1910 the population of the United States grew 138 percent, but the number of doctors grew by 153 percent.

A relationship existed between the oversupply of physicians and the economic uncertainty that many of them experienced. Too many doctors enabled the public to control the price for medical services. Some practitioner could almost always be found who would underbid his brethren; hence, the ever-present item of the fee bill on the Nashville Medical Society's agenda.

For so many physicians to earn at least part of a livelihood by the practice of medicine, the income of some of them had to remain depressed. Thus large numbers of doctors in late nineteenth century America also farmed, tended store, held forth from a pulpit on Sunday morning, or taught school. Part-time practitioners tended to resist codes of ethics, licensing laws, and other public and private regulation.

Unregulated growth and competition marked many social and economic activities in the Gilded Age. Railroads laid track, entrepreneurs penetrated markets, farmers expanded their acreage, all without regard to long-term profitability. Too many physicians per patient was a comparable phenomenon. In medicine, as in business, ruinous price wars followed.

The quality of medical education was fraught with implications for physicians' financial standing: making medical schools more difficult to enter and to complete would decrease the number of practitioners and raise the prospects of those who won the diploma. But the issue of improved educational standards, while it included questions of economics, went beyond them. The achievement of professional status and authority by physicians required that they become better trained, presenting credentials and producing results manifestly superior to those offered by sellers of patent medicine, homeopathists, and all the rest.

An era of discovery about the nature and causes of some major diseases was indeed underway. Doctors divided over the bedside uses of new laboratory findings and diagnostic tools, debates heard in the Nashville Medical Society and in the pages of the *Nashville Journal of Medicine and Surgery*. Many of the new advances, whether in antiseptic surgery, immunology, or therapeutics, came after false starts. Robert Koch's premature announcement in 1890 of a cure for tuberculosis was one such debacle.

The concepts and techniques of bacteriology nonetheless hastened the transformation of medicine into a scientific discipline. The refinement of antisepsis in the 1870s, the discovery of specific pathogens in the 1880s, and progress in chemotherapy in the 1890s and after 1900 resulted from work by European and American bacteriologists. Even though there was a time lag between gains in knowledge of pathology and the treatment of disease, the momentum of scientific medicine would be fully apparent by the 1910s and 1920s.

Medical schools offered the logical mechanism for transmitting the new findings about disease. Early in the twentieth century, educational reformers insisted that science, represented by and embodied in teaching hospitals and laboratories, was the substance and goal of medical school. The achievement of control over medical education and licensing, with the assistance of the state, enabled physicians to diminish competition, raise professional qualifications, and attain unprecedented public regard. Organized medicine's drive to that success gave it the power it enjoyed through most of the rest of the twentieth century. In Nashville, one can see that great national story writ small.

THE ONGOING STRUGGLE TO ORGANIZE

A city medical society had been intermittently active in Nashville during the 1820s, 1830s, and 1840s, being reconstituted in 1858. A county society formed in 1853, but did not appear again in the antebellum historical record. No medical organization was visible during the Civil War. In 1866 the Nashville Medical Society reassembled, remained active for three years, then disappeared until the epidemic year of 1873. On August 14, 1874 a group of prominent physicians reorganized the society, adopting with minor amendments the old constitution. At the first regular meeting, Dr. Thomas O. Summers, Jr., called attention to the necessity for eliciting interest, the lack of which had thwarted attempts at organization.

The defense of doctors' economic interests became, once again, one of the society's goals, no doubt a priority one in this time of national depression. An *ad hoc* committee reported that

> "Some persons living in Nashville had owed doctors' bills for twenty years, and had never paid a dime, [but] as doctors had to buy meat, bread, coal, and other necessities of life it was certainly right that all doctors' fees should be paid when it was known that the person was able to pay them but wouldn't. . . ."

Acting on the committee's recommendation, the society resolved to make charges uniform and reaffirmed that fees were due at the time service was rendered, with office visits ("*especially* venereal cases") to be paid in cash. All doctors, whether members of the society or not, were requested to present to its secretary the name and address of

The University of Nashville

In a speech delivered in 1837, President Philip Lindsley of the University of Nashville expressed the hope of establishing faculties of law and medicine there. The idea languished until the early 1850s when Drs. William K. Bowling and John Berrien Lindsley formed a medical club, which later became the faculty that Lindsley's father had proposed. While retaining complete autonomy, it called itself the medical department of the University, and leased facilities there. This group comprised, in addition to the two founders,

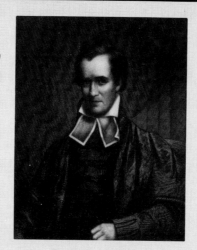

Dr. Phillip Lindsley

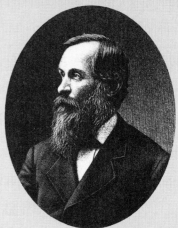

Dr. John Berrien Lindsley

Drs. William Briggs, A. H. Buchanan, Paul F. Eve, Robert M. Porter, John M. Watson, and Charles K. Winston.

The first session opened in November, 1851, one hundred twenty one students enrolled and thirty three graduated the following year. The acme was reached in 1859-60, when more than four hundred fifty matriculated. In the number of alumni, the school ranked second among medical colleges in the nation. Two courses of four months duration were required for graduation. Summer courses, described by department

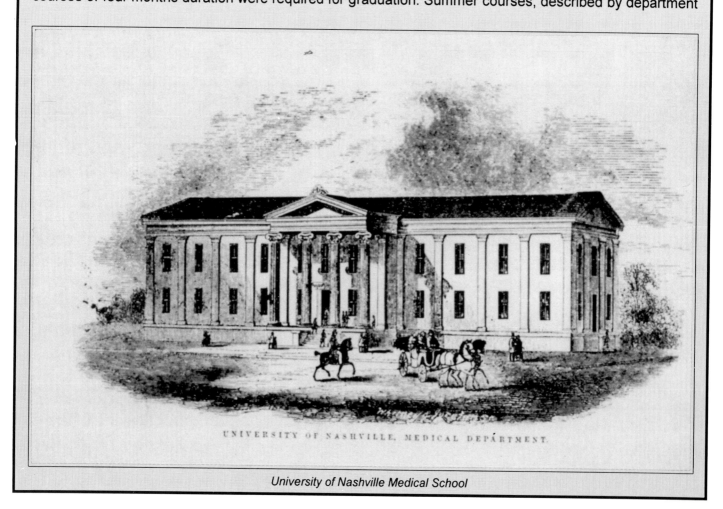

UNIVERSITY OF NASHVILLE, MEDICAL DEPARTMENT.

University of Nashville Medical School

literature as "practical in character," were inaugurated in 1855, but not required.

The investment was a profitable one for the physician investors, and the school competed successfully with older established ones in Louisville and Philadelphia. Between 1851 and 1880, nearly seven thousand students came to the University of Nashville to study medicine, and some two thousand two hundred graduated. In that period two of its faculty, Drs. Bowling and Eve, were elected president of the American Medical Association, and five others served as vice presidents. No other college in the nation could match that record.

Perhaps it was as good a medical education as was then available in the old Southwest. Yet Dr. Daniel Drake and many others despaired of the quality of students enrolled in proprietary schools, where faculty-owners collected fees for the courses of lectures they gave. He wrote, "Their ranks are filled up with recruits deficient in abilities or requirements . . . [They are] too stupid for the bar, too immoral for the pulpit."

The department never recovered from the disruption of the war and enrollment dwindled to an average of 150 a year. On April 21, 1874, the medical faculty entered into an agreement with the new Vanderbilt University, which provided that students matriculating at the latter should receive its diploma, but those attending the University of Nashville would be graduated as before. As Vanderbilt's prestige grew, it drew the greater number of enrollees, and the two institutions dissolved their medical partnership in 1895.

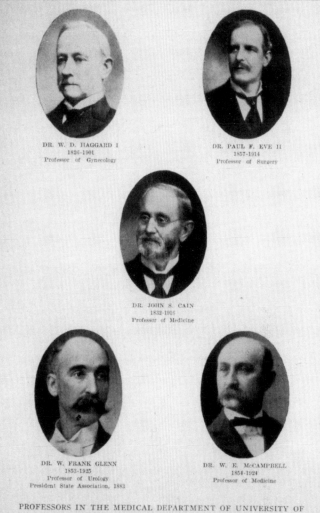

DR. W. D. HAGGARD I
1826-1901
Professor of Gynecology

DR. PAUL F. EVE II
1857-1914
Professor of Surgery

DR. JOHN S. CAIN
1832-1916
Professor of Medicine

DR. W. FRANK GLENN
1853-1925
Professor of Urology
President State Association, 1882

DR. W. E. McCAMPBELL
1854-1921
Professor of Medicine

PROFESSORS IN THE MEDICAL DEPARTMENT OF UNIVERSITY OF TENNESSEE WHEN AT NASHVILLE

Professors in the Medical Department of the University of Tennessee: Dr. William D. Haggard, professor of gynecology; Dr. Paul F. Eve, Jr., professor of surgery; Dr. John S. Cain, professor of medicine; Dr. W. Frank Glenn, professor of urology; Dr. W. E. McCampbell, professor of medicine

Shelby Medical College

Following the initial success of the University of Nashville's medical department, four other physicians entered into the sweepstakes to train doctors for profit. In 1857 Drs. John H. Callendar, John P. Ford, and Thomas L. Maddin, and John Shelby established the Shelby Medical College. They had hoped to make it the medical department of a proposed "Central University" of the Methodist Episcopal Church South, an institution that materialized as Vanderbilt University after the war. Shelby Medical College stood on the site of the present-day United States Customs House.

As in most schools of the day, there was no clinical or laboratory experience, the diploma attested to no special competence, and no one was bound to honor it. Nashville's medical schools, popular, celebrated, and financially successful, provided that anyone could practice medicine.

Enrollment rose from eighty five that first year to one hundred twenty in 1859. With the coming of the war, Shelby Medical College closed its doors, and its buildings were seized for hospitals.

The University of Tennessee Medical Department

In the summer of 1876, Drs. Duncan Eve and W. F. Glenn organized the Nashville Medical College. The first session opened the following March, with a part-time faculty (like all schools of the time) comprising Paul F. Eve, T. B. Buchanan, and William K. Bowling. The first class graduated in 1878.

The following year the trustees of the University of Tennessee proposed to adopt the enterprise as the medical department of that institution. From 1879-89, the student body averaged 171 enrolled each year and 61 new physicians graduated annually. Entrance requirements were nominal, and the course of instruction covered a period of two years (as was generally common). As many as one hundred diplomas were given out at some commencements.

The year before Flexner's study appeared, the local medical profession helped sponsor the consolidation of the University of Nashville's medical department and that of the University of Tennessee. The new school operated under a joint name, but by 1912 morale under its faculty had collapsed, and many doctor-teachers

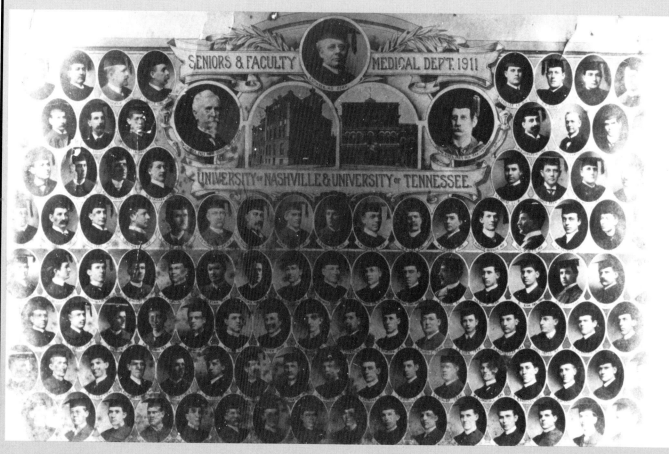

Faculty and seniors, the Medical Department of the University of Nashville and the University of Tennessee, Class of 1911. This was the last class to graduate before the dissolution of the institution.

offered their services to Vanderbilt. Students followed, and Vanderbilt grew in size, though quality was still another matter.

In mid-summer, 1911, Chancellor James H. Kirkland of Vanderbilt announced that the University of Nashville would cease medical teaching altogether, and the University of Tennessee's department of medicine would find a new home city, first in Knoxville, then Memphis.

Vanderbilt University School of Medicine

The influential Flexner Report of 1910, underwritten by the Carnegie Foundation, had lambasted Vanderbilt's medical school for lax admissions, high rate of dropouts, and foul dissecting rooms. Still, Flexner concluded, it was the best of a bad lot in the South and thus worth upgrading.

Chancellor Kirkland understood the demands on his school. The University would have to expand its hospital to provide for research and bedside teaching. It would have to find the means to hire full-time faculty and not depend on doctors who earned most of their living treating patients outside.

All this required vast sums of money. The chancellor won the interest of the General Education Board—the prosaic name under which John D. Rockefeller dispensed portions of his fortune. From about 1910 to the 1940s, the agency became the largest single supporter of

Professors in the Vanderbilt University Medical Department at the time of its separation from the University of Nashville, 1895: Dr. Richard Douglas, professor of gynecology and abdominal surgery; Dr. John J. Witherspoon, professor of medicine; Dr. William L. Dudley, dean and professor of chemistry; Dr. Thomas Menees, professor of obstetrics; Dr. George H. Price, professor of physiology and diseases of the ear, nose, and throat.

medical education in the nation, and Vanderbilt was among the greatest beneficiaries. With an initial gift of $150,000, the university was able to acquire the former properties of the University of Nashville on Rutledge Hill, owned by George Peabody College for Teachers. There Chancellor Kirkland hoped to build a new Vanderbilt Medical Department. (As part of the deal, Peabody agreed to exchange this property for acreage owned by Vanderbilt on Twenty-first Avenue, South, southeast of its main campus.)

The new buildings were the least of it, however; to keep pace with rising standards Vanderbilt had to impose admission standards of at least one year of college. In 1914 enrollment dropped drastically, from 100 to 19. Fees plummeted, too.

As income dropped costs went up, for hospital facilities and the salaries of full-time, teachers. Vanderbilt faced a choice—make a major investment in the medical school, or leave the field.

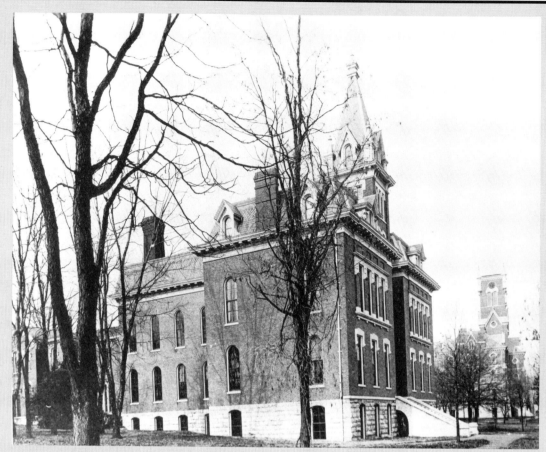

Science Hall (foreground) and Main Building, Vanderbilt University, early 1890s

Four millions of Rockefeller's money, awarded late in 1919, made an entirely new campus possible. In 1921, there came three million for endowment, half from the GEB, half from the Carnegie Foundation. In the fall of 1925, the first class arrived at the new hospital and classroom, located adjacent to the University's main campus. They studied with a legendary faculty recruited by Dean Canby Robinson. Among these were Drs. Alfred Blalock, Barney Brooks, Sidney Burwell, Ernest W. Goodpasture, Tinsley Harrison, Rudolph H. Kampmeier, Waller S. Leathers, Hugh Morgan, and John Youmans. Several had ties to Rockefeller charities; even more were graduates of or had held appointments at Johns Hopkins School of Medicine.

Meharry Medical College

Meharry's parent institution, Central Tennessee College, began as a primary school sponsored by the Methodist Church after the Civil War. For several years it was a college in name only, but soon students qualified for courses in advanced subjects.

President John Braden attributed the idea for a medical department to a bright student who asked if the college could furnish such facilities. To open them, the Reverend Braden recruited two war veterans, one a Northern man, the other a Southerner. George W. Hubbard, from New Hampshire, had come

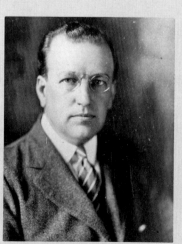

Dr. Canby Robinson

to Nashville with the Christian Commission, attached to the Union's Army of the Cumberland. Dr. William J. Sneed, a Tennessean and former Confederate Army surgeon, came to the college in 1875 to offer the first basic courses. The following year he and Hubbard, who had just received his M.D. at Vanderbilt, opened the Meharry Medical Department near present-day Lafayette Street in the Trimble Bottom neighborhood. The name honored five brothers, prosperous farmers of Ohio and Indiana from an abolitionist family, who gave the first major gift to start the department.

Dentistry, pharmacy, and nursing were added to the curriculum before the end of the century. The Flexner Report urged philanthropists to let most of the nation's black medical schools expire, due to their low standards, and put resources behind just two: the one at Howard University, and Meharry. In part to assure that such investment would not be encumbered by its declining parent school, Meharry separated itself from

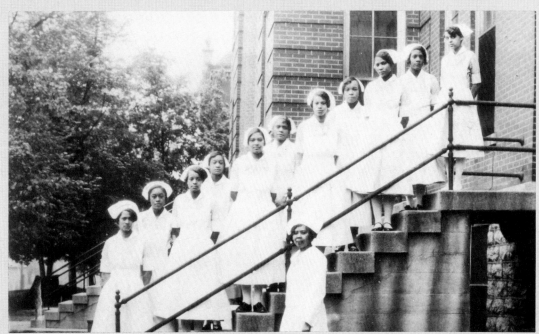

Nurse training class at Meharry, 1918

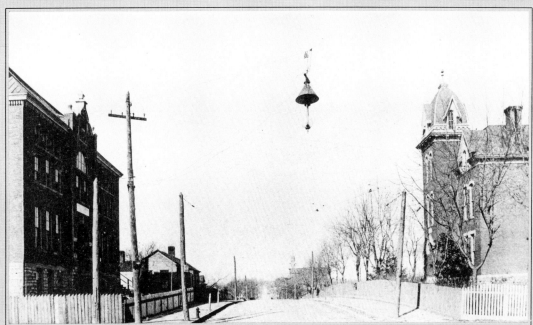

Central Tennessee College and its Meharry Medical Department (right side of street), forerunner of Meharry Medical College

Central Tennessee College and from Methodist control in 1915.

The General Education Board hoped Meharry would merge with Fisk University. The trustees gently declined, but the GEB physically associated the two schools by building Meharry a new north Nashville campus across the street from the university. As at Fisk, Meharry students and faculty expressed hopes for an increase in blacks in leadership positions, and many Meharry teaching faculty took leave for specialty training, hoping to return to head departments.

With the closure of the University of Nashville and the departure of the University of Tennessee's medical program, the city was left with two schools for the training of doctors, Meharry and Vanderbilt. A summary of their modern history is given in part two of this essay, beginning on page 109.

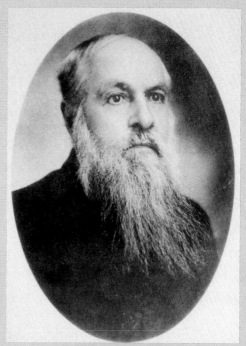

Dr. George W. Hubbard

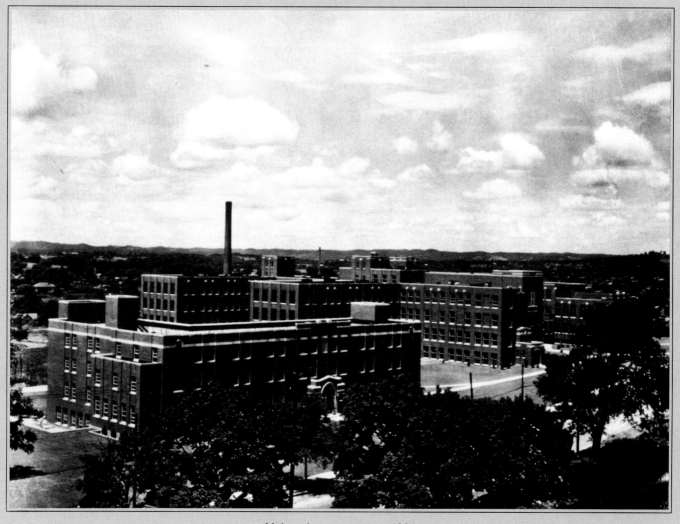

Meharry's new campus, 1931

every debtor; none was to be attended until the bill was paid.

Enforcement of standards—including uniform fees, the provisions of the American Medical Association's Code of Ethics, and more stringent requirements in medical schools—became a major theme of the *Nashville Journal of Medicine and Surgery*'s editorial page in these years. From its founding in 1851, the journal upheld the ideal of a profession that set and controlled the qualifications of its own members without intervention by third parties. This position reflected the views of publisher William K. Bowling. In the summer of 1875—following his election to the presidency of the AMA—Bowling resigned from the *Journal* and conveyed its affairs (presumably by sale) to Drs. William T. Briggs and Thomas O. Summers, Jr. In January, 1877 the ownership passed into control of Drs. William L. Nichol and Charles Briggs.

Nichol and Briggs differed markedly from Bowling when it came to a self-regulating profession. Their flagship editorial declared:

> "We shall strive to spread the belief that State legislation for regulating the practice of medicine is the only available method for purging the profession free from those parasites for whose misdeeds we are so heavily responsible."

Until such a law was enacted, the *Journal* urged that the Tennessee State Medical Society become a judicial council and "bring before its tribunal all the numerous offenders." Nichol and Briggs claimed to witness daily violations of the AMA Code of Ethics:

> "Here we see a physician seeking his neighbor's patient and offering his services at a lower fee or *gratis*. There again, another who boasts of his professional skill or knowledge. Here one who seeks newspaper renown and unblushingly hands the account of some wonderful operation to the local editor. Here another who regrets that he did not offer his services *gratis*, in order to prevent his personal enemy from getting the fee."

AN EFFORT AT SELF-REGULATION

This proposed regulatory role was soon tried. In June, 1878, fifty physicians organized the Davidson County Medical Society. As other local associations of doctors had done, this group offered a forum where members could read and hear essays and discuss cases with fellow practitioners. However, the main feature of the society, and evidently the main purpose for which it was begun, was to sponsor a board of supervisors. This panel would adjudicate all professional misdemeanors and irregularities, presumably including those that Drs. Nichol and Briggs lamented. These combative editors looked forward to the "medical court martial" of a "number of prominent physicians who have fallen by the wayside. . . .Abuse of professional privileges have [sic] of late grown so flagrant that it is almost a disgrace to belong to the profession."

For unknown reasons, the plan failed. In his valedictory address to the society in 1879, Dr. W. C. Blackman, its president, referred to the "everlasting perhaps," spoken of by Dr. William Osler, and the limitations of medical intervention, which Dr. Paul F. Eve insisted should make physicians slow to judge one another. Blackman's speech actually proposed greater rather than less passivity:

> "It is impossible to have each member be just what he ought to be; there are difficulties which prevent it being done. . . .Although we may hear of some short coming in a neighbor, without a thorough knowledge of all the facts and motive of the offender, we cannot make a case, and to attempt to bring the guilty to judgment only ends in our injury. . .I can only suggest that each of us zealously endeavor to do right and not spend his time seeking to pull the beams from others' eyes."

The *Nashville Journal of Medicine and Surgery* promised to report any investigation undertaken by the society, but none was ever published. Indeed, no further word of the group was heard for seven years.

POPULAR SKEPTICISM

Openness and candor about their theoretical differences scarcely encouraged the public to accept regular physicians' claims to a monopoly on scientific validity. When printed in local newspapers, medical society debates revealed the gap between professional aspiration and physicians' powerlessness before most diseases. Worse still, here were doctors in open and flagrant disagreement. In a discussion of bloodletting before the Nashville Medical Society on December 16, 1875, Drs. G. W. Currey and J. W. Morton (the City Health Officer, 1874-76) argued for the efficacy of the procedure. Dr. W. Frank Glenn retorted that it had become an almost forgotten art and should be "buried in oblivion."

When speakers before the society denounced other kinds of practitioners, their attacks reinforced the image of one economic group competing against another, an image suggested by such newspaper story captions as "Reopening of the War Between the Doctors and Druggists / A Scorching Review of Business Relations." Some in the medical fraternity genuinely believed that pharmacists threatened their incomes. Speaking to the Nashville Medical Society in 1875, Dr. G. W. Currey accused the city's druggist so dispensing doctors' formulae at reduced prices:

> "The present system has resulted in the springing up of a lot of little drug stores on nearly every corner in the city, and many of them depend almost solely upon their prescription trade. . . .Each druggist has become a kind of sub-doctor, who competes with you daily, and prescribes and treats more cases of venereal disease than any of you, and to whom you have unsolicited, of your own free will and accord, exposed your hands."

The apothecaries' shelves stocked another bane of Nashville doctors, patent medicine. Lacking ownership of their prescriptions, physicians permitted druggists to collect fees that should have been theirs; lacking authority over patent medicine, they could do nothing to prevent sick people from treating themselves for the price of a nostrum. Patent medicine companies also served as "sub-doctors": they not only sold drugs but published health guides and dispensed medical advice by mail. Playing upon the widespread public distrust of medicine, they provided the beleaguered physician still more competition.

Not all the professional relations between physicians and pharmacists were inimical. Dr. Van S. Lindsley, a president of the Nashville Medical Society, told that body in 1874 that druggists daily receive prescriptions from doctors for quack remedies. Some doctors evidently entered into agreements with a particular apothecary and directed patients solely to him.

Realizing the self-injury done by public revelations of both competition and collusion, the Nashville Medical Society in January, 1876, excluded newspaper reporters from its sessions. Although apparently active through the

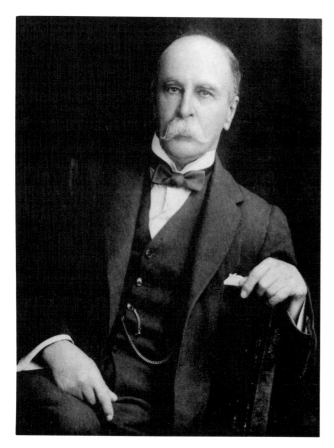

Sir William Osler

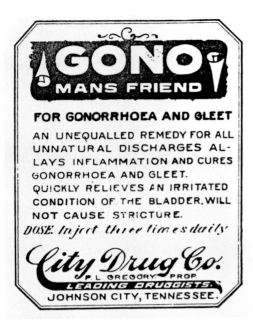

Patent medicines, such as this one manufactured in Johnson City, Tennessee, enabled druggists to compete vigorously with physicians.

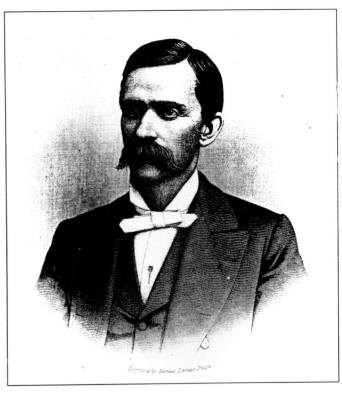

Dr. Van S. Lindsley

election of Dr. James Plunket as president in 1877, the city society thereafter sank from view and evidently remained in abeyance for almost ten years.

The year 1879 witnessed an attempt to form another city-based society, the "Nashville Academy of Medicine." This group set forth an ambitious program of clinical reports and papers, including lectures in medicine, obstetrics, surgery, and other subjects. Although the Academy secured a meeting hall, it apparently fared no better than previous such groups in sustaining interest and commitment of members. The *Nashville Journal of Medicine and Surgery* noted that the city had been "peculiarly unfortunate in our local organizations," attributing the numerous failures to "the great interval between meetings" and the lack of "proper pablum" for discussion.

The continual failure of medical societies meant the continual failure of self-regulation by physicians. The regular physicians' search for social and economic security was inseparable from honest outrage at the abuses they perceived. Worst among these, in their view, were unqualified practitioners.

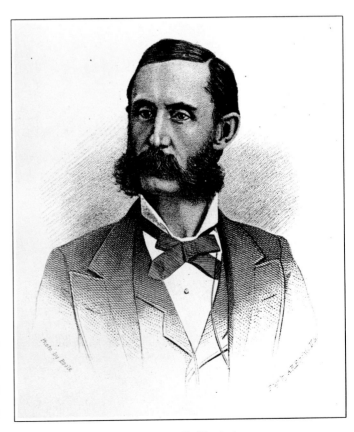

Dr. James D. Plunket

Nashville's Medical Societies; A Roster

As in other cities throughout America, Nashville medical societies experienced periodic suspensions and reorganizations. The *Nashville Journal of Medicine and Surgery* observed in 1879 that the city had been "peculiarly unfortunate" in the number of unsuccessful attempts by doctors to join together. A discussion of some of the reasons for those failures, prior to the establishment of the Nashville Academy of Medicine, can be found in the text, particularly Chapter Four.

1821
unnamed society organizes to regulate fees

1828
first mention in the historical record of the Nashville Medical Society

1830
Tennessee State Medical Association forms

1830-44
historical record gives no mention of Nashville Medical Society

1844
Nashville Medical Society reappears in historical record

1853
Davidson County Medical Society organizes, but does not reappear in the antebellum historical record

1853-58
historical record gives no mention of Nashville Medical Society

June 1858
Nashville Medical Society reorganizes

1862-65
Nashville Medical Society suspends for duration of the war

1865
Nashville Medical Society revives

1868-73
historical record gives no mention of Nashville Medical Society

1872
Edgefield Medical Society organizes

1874
Nashville Medical Society reorganizes

1877-86
Nashville Medical Society disappears from historical record

1878
Davidson County Medical Society reorganizes

1879
attempt to organize a "Nashville Academy of Medicine" fails

1880-86
historical record gives no mention of Davidson County Medical Society

1886
Nashville Academy of Medicine forms
Davidson County Medical Society reorganizes

1889
Nashville Obstetrical and Gynecological Society organizes

1893
Nashville Academy of Medicine and Davidson County Medical Society merge

1898
Medico-Chirurgical Club of Nashville forms

1903
black physicians form a Medico-Chirurgical Society

1903
Negro Medical Congress of Tennessee is organized, later called the Volunteer State Medical Association

1903-07
black physicians' group apparently undergoes several reorganizations; takes the name Rock City Academy of Medicine and Surgery, then the R. F. Boyd Medical Society

1963
Tennessee State Medical Association changes name to Tennessee Medical Association

On scientific grounds regular physicians assailed homeopathists, whose presence in the city was visible in the Davidson County Homeopathic Society, organized in 1870. Dr. John W. Maddin, Sr., devoted his presidential address before the revived Nashville Academy of Medicine in 1886 to a withering attack upon homeopathy, labeling it the "miserable spawn of a disordered mind." Like regular medicine, however, homeopathy represented a rational system, and many of its practitioners were trained in large, well-capitalized medical schools. Homeopathy was particularly popular among socially prominent and upper-income families, providing formidable economic competition against regular medicine.

The medical profession in Nashville, as throughout the nation, divided over the issue of whether its members might consult with homeopathists, a practice forbidden by the AMA Code of Ethics. When in 1882 the New York State medical society called for repeal of this provision, the *Nashville Journal of Medicine and Surgery* blasted this action. But in a rebuttal, Dr. J. S. Nowlin of Nashville noted the popularity of homeopathy and the futility of attempting to exclude its practitioners from professional and fraternal association. The presence in Nashville of several regularly-trained physicians who practiced the homeopathic regimen demonstrated, despite Dr. Maddin's ferocity, the occasional convergence of the two systems.

Competition from other doctors trained like themselves created hurdles for every ambitious regular practitioner of late nineteenth century Nashville. To win economic, professional, and social advantage, such physicians sought ways to distinguish themselves from their brethren. Appointment to the faculty of a medical school gave a physician additional presumptive authority. The regular profession in Nashville sought to borrow the public esteem attached to education in the "Athens of the South," and to a notable extent it succeeded. Reporters sometimes refer to local physicians as "our medical faculty." When they finally achieved an enduring organization, Nashville's regular doctors incorporated as the "Academy of Medicine."

Some successful physicians opened small proprietary hospitals that served as medical boarding houses for well-to-do clientele. One such was the Nashville Infirmary. An 1880 advertisement claimed that "the faculty of the Medical Department of the University of Nashville and Vanderbilt University constitute the medical and surgical staff."

Specialization was another means of differentiating oneself from other physicians. Perhaps the foremost new specialty in the post-Civil War years was surgery, which enjoyed a spectacular rise in esteem and achievement with improvements in antisepsis. Surgeons soon organized their own medical societies that helped distinguish their calling.

The creation of organizations by other kinds of specialists served to validate their skill and training when the devalued credential of a medical diploma could not. The Nashville Obstetrical and Gynecological Society, organized in 1889, comprised members of the medical faculties and owners of the prominent private hospitals. The Edgefield Medical Society, presumably comprising practitioners in that affluent suburb, formed in 1872. Specialist societies could also serve as winnowing devices for an over-crowded profession. The Medico-Chirurgical Club of Nashville, established in 1898, limited its membership to sixteen.

The success of specialist societies compared with the struggle of non-specialist organizations can be explained by the advantages they gave to members. The additional credential of specialist designation—awarded by societies in this era before hospital residencies and certification—was presumably negotiable for higher fees. Belonging to the medical society added little monetary or social value to one's diploma. Specialists may have had fewer areas of therapeutic disagreement, while groups like the Nashville and Davidson County medical societies were riven with discord. Finally, specialists had a professional goal to serve the promotion of their own authority.

ENTERING THE PUBLIC REALM

Growing acceptance of the germ theory gave physicians in general an opportunity to claim authority in public health and, thereby, an entree into the political process. Asking for the state's action against incompetent doctors—their competitors and professional foes—physicians offered to act in turn as public guardians on a whole host of health issues.

The initial cooperation between organized medicine and public policymakers came in the area of sanitation. The Nashville Medical Society's role in creating a city board of health in 1866 gave the regular physicians a visible role whenever public health issues arose. Within a few years that board dissolved, and the medical society also lapsed.

It can hardly be coincidental that the Nashville Medical Society reappeared in the aftermath of the cholera epidemic of 1873. The disaster also caused the city to reestablish the board of health.

Widespread disagreement existed about the cause of cholera, the mode of its transmission, and the most effective means to combat it. This confusion openly revealed itself at the Nashville meeting of the American Association for the Advancement of Science in 1877, when Mrs. H. K. Ingram of Edgefield—in the first paper ever read before the AAAS by a woman—proposed that cholera germs could be killed by concussion and called for the explosion of heavy charges of gunpowder day and night during the epidemic season.

At the nation's centenary, Nashville had the highest death rate of any city in the United States and, of those cities reporting, the fifth highest in the world. Its poorly-drained streets, open sewers, and foul garbage heaps appalled visitors. Privies and kitchen pipes at the State Penitentiary, located a mile west of the Public Square, seeped into open streams flowing through town. Wells, even in the fashionable residential sections, were often contaminated. The purity of the city's water supply seemed doubtful, since four cemeteries, a public dump, a tannery, and innumerable privies stood on the Cumberland River only a short distance above the water system's intake pipes.

Influential parties pointed to the causal connection between filth and disease in the city. The *Daily American*, the morning newspaper, urged that sanitarians' advice be heeded and the board of health invested with police powers to close contaminated wells and abolish all surface toilets. Its editorial page repeatedly called for a thorough system of sewage disposal. Sanitary improvements ought to become an issue in mayoral races, it insisted, and it urged candidates to propose practical plans to alleviate the constant threats of cholera, diphtheria, typhoid, and other plagues.

Although new scientific ideas, especially the germ theory, were debated in the Nashville Medical Society, their implications for public policy were not. Regardless, preventive medicine could not yet serve as an organizing and sustaining principle for a medical society. Its approach, in contrast to curative or elective medicine, stressed cooperative impulses and collective action while doctors, by and large, remained highly competitive and radically individualistic.

Nonetheless, society leadership passed into the hands of a sanitarian when Dr. James Plunket became president in 1877. Other heads of the organization—Dr. Thomas Menees (1866-68) and Thomas A. Atchison (1887) addressed the public on the importance of cleanliness in the prevention of disease. This trio and other medical society members led the movement for a comprehensive sewerage system and a pure water supply and served as officers and members of the Board of Health. When they spoke out for the health advantages of a cleaner city, they conjoined the twin authorities of the public health board and organized medicine.

Winning popular support for this sanitary science, these physicians put state power behind the prescriptions that were medicine's most effective regimen of the time—clean streets, pure water, wholesome food. From that position they sought legislative and regulatory aid in raising professional standards, which the medical societies, acting alone, had been unable to accomplish.

THE CONSOLIDATION OF AUTHORITY

Nashville physicians failed to achieve a lasting organization during this period because they were unable to decide whether the medical society should be inclusive or exclusive. The former strategy would open membership to all practitioners, regardless of qualifications; the latter would set qualifications relative to education and conformity with professional rules.

The membership rule that the Nashville Medical Society set in 1858 sought that end. But its rigid application would have kept the group a small, elite one, vulnerable to distraction, lack of interest, and dissolution.

Ultimately, educational credentials—as implied in the 1858 rule—offered a way to accomplish that exclusion. First, however, the physicians such as those organized in the Nashville Medical Society and like groups around the nation had to gain monopoly over the content of medical college curricula and institute there a medicine based on laboratory findings and patient observation. To win that monopoly would take state support, which in turn required that doctors demonstrate a medicine that worked. The great age of prevention in the late nineteenth century gave them this opportunity.

For half a century Nashville's various short-lived medical societies had spoken for the aspirations of a certain kind of physician, one well-trained in a reputable medical school. However, the presence of too many practitioners—some poorly educated, some fraudulent, some willing to negotiate fees with patients—diminished the advantages that should naturally have accrued to the doctor with thorough training. It therefore became necessary for organized medicine to eliminate the bottom tier—quacks, pretenders, men with too little learning—and raise the middle segment through improved educational standards.

By the mid-1880s legislators were expressing considerable interest in protecting the public from medical fraud and abuse. In his valedictory address to the Tennessee State Medical Association in 1874, Dr. J. J. Abernathy, the president, proposed the creation of a State Medical Commission to "examine every physician within the state, issuing certificates of qualification to such only, as in their judgment, are deserving." Although the state medical society experienced its own organizing and recruiting difficulties throughout this period, it persisted in its call for the creation of a board of physicians to examine candidates and issue licenses. The slowness of the General Assembly to act on such a measure—first proposed in 1803—was attributed by the society's historian to popular opposition to "class legislation," a Jacksonian interpretation and one that assumes the public had little expectation of physicians.

Many doctors, even well-educated ones, argued against a licensing law. In the face of the opposition, a committee of the state society chaired by Dr. J. S. Cain (subsequently president of the Nashville Academy of Medicine) drew up a bill, urged its passage in the General Assembly, and

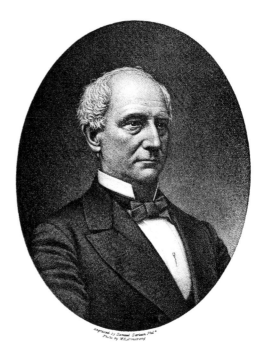

Dr. Thomas Menees

achieved that success in 1889. This law provided for a State Board of Medical Examiners comprising six members, two from each of Tennessee's Grand Divisions.

To the regular physicians' dismay, the original language was amended to require that the board include representation from the "three schools of medicine, viz.: Allopath, Homeopath, and Eclectic." The statue embodied the state society's essential aim, however: before practicing medicine in Tennessee, one was required to obtain a certificate from the board. It provided a potential means of eliminating quacks and pretenders. It also gave doctors in the Tennessee society a political agenda: the amendment of the law to narrow, then eliminate approval for homeopathic and eclectic physicians. To influence this application of state power, the organization of doctors, formerly a desideratum, became imperative.

Other educational, political, and economic goals of physicians needed state action. In 1878 the *Nashville Journal of Medicine and Surgery* urged the General Assembly to legalize dissection, utilizing bodies of criminals and paupers. The *Journal* later endorsed a bill to provide for the registration of births, marriages, and deaths in Tennessee. Acts to regulate dentistry and pharmacy passed in 1891 and 1893, respectively, and restrictions were placed on itinerant physicians, long reviled in society debates and the medical press.

THE NASHVILLE ACADEMY OF MEDICINE FORMS

A medical society with an unbroken existence, the Nashville Academy of Medicine and Surgery, was at last established in Nashville in the spring of 1886. On the evening of April 15, a number of physicians met in the office of Professor T. J. Dodd at the Watkins Institute, Dr. Newton G. Tucker in the chair. Elected president that evening was Dr. John W. Maddin, Sr. In his inaugural address at the organizational meeting on April 22, Dr. Maddin spoke of medicine's emerging relations with public policy:

"We are closely related to the body politic through our system of medical jurisprudence, in the administration of civil and criminal law. Life insurance, involving the laws of longevity as affected by heredity and diathesis, call for a skilled prognosis as well as a scientific application of the methods of physical diagnosis. Municipal legislation calls us to positions of health officers, with the obligation of the trusts of public sanitation of dwellings, school houses, factories, of nuisances, of food adulteration and purity and freshness of vegetables, meats, and milk, the prevention of contagious diseases by vaccination disinfection; the registration of births and deaths, the causes of mortality, and how to lessen the death rate; the causes and prevention of epidemics."

Within a few days of the founding of the Nashville Academy of Medicine, the Davidson County Medical Society (inactive since 1880) was reorganized. At its first meeting, Dr. J. B. W. Nowlin was elected president. There are "many things we might discuss," he told his colleagues,

"matters of great importance to us doctors, but of more importance to our county and city. As an example, with our population of 60,000 to 70,000 in the city proper and half so many more in the county, we have no first-class hospital. . ."

Dr. Thomas A. Atchison served as president of the Nashville Academy of Medicine in its second year, succeeded in 1888 by Dr. W. A. Atchison. Dr. William D. Haggard (himself president in 1892) chronicled this early history before an 1891 meeting. He recalled that interest had once again flagged in 1888, a session that fall attended by only four members. Those four, pondering how to revive participation, decided to pray over the matter. From that time, Dr. Haggard told his listeners, the Academy had prospered. He did not know, he added, that this result was attributable to the prayer, "but probably it was not."

The morale of the Academy rose and its treasury grew as a result of the meeting of the American Medical Association in Nashville in 1890, at which Dr. William T. Briggs was elected president. Just prior to the AMA's meeting, delegates from 55 of the nation's medical schools convened in Tennessee's capital to discuss reformation in the training of doctors. An association of such institutions had formed in 1876 and been abandoned. Now those assembled revived the National Association of Medical Colleges, subsequently called the Association of American Medical Colleges, and prescribed a set of standards that member institutions had to meet.

By the winter of 1891 the Nashville Academy of Medicine was sufficiently confident of its future to rent "for a term of years" new quarters in the Mill Block, 621 Church Street. Its program in honor of taking possession of the new hall included two addresses that focused on the social and political status of Nashville physicians. Academy members assembled every Thursday night. Business matters were reserved to the first meeting in the month. Other sessions were devoted to the reading and discussion of essays and reports of clinical cases. Some evenings evidently passed in desultory talk. "Cigarette smoking has been discussed," one source noted, "and it is now in contemplation to take up the subject of wearing mourning for the dead."

Yet, in due time, the Academy was called again to set public service as a central purpose for its being. In his presidential address in 1897, Dr. Arch M. Trawick quoted former President Grover Cleveland's query to the New York Academy of Medicine: Had members of the profession in their onward march left behind their sense of civic obligation and their interest in the general public welfare? In reply, Dr. Trawick told Nashville doctors:

> "A conscience involving a sense of personal obligation to do one's whole duty is as much a necessity for citizenship as for the narrower spheres of domestic and professional life."

The Tennessee licensing act, the call for a public hospital, the key role in the organization of the nation's medical colleges—in all of this Nashville doctors took an unprecedented public role. But physicians' "consolidation of authority"—the phrase is Paul Starr's—would await the coming of the social reforms associated with the Progressive era. Like many of those reforms, the uplift and unification of the profession would be ambiguous in its outcomes. Therapeutic advances would establish science at the heart of medicine, and require the training of doctors in arcane and specialized fields about which patients could know little. The gaining of a monopoly over educational standards and licensing eliminated real abuses of the past, but there followed a decreased supply of doctors, a maldistribution of medical services, and increased costs for them.

With the merger in 1893 of the Nashville Academy of Medicine and the Davidson County Medical Society, local doctors celebrated an unalloyed accomplishment: an enduring organization after 70 years of confused, intermittent attempts. Although still claiming only a fraction of them as members, the Nashville Academy of Medicine made physicians' collective presence felt in the opening years of the twentieth century.

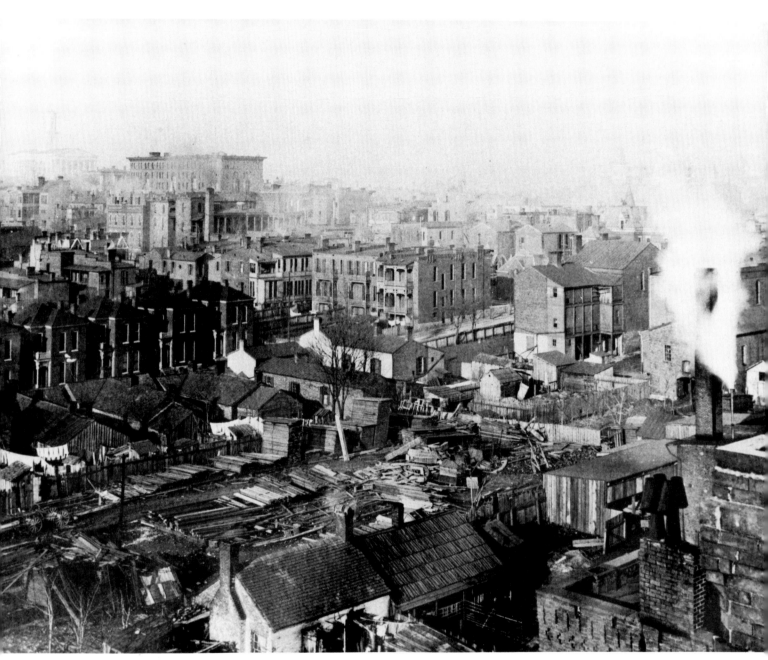

Nashville's polluted air and primitive public sanitation aroused the concern of many
physicians at the turn of the last century. This view is south of Broad Street.

Chapter Five

PHYSICIANS AND THE
ERA OF REFORM

"Does the twentieth century begin on the first day of 1900 or the first day of 1901?" The question stimulated much discussion in the editorial columns and from the pulpits of Nashville as the new century approached. Content to leave the matter unsettled, hosts and hostesses lit the porch lamps on the snowbound evening of December 31, 1899, and their guests braved the streets to reach the laden tables and decorated halls.

Unsettled, too, as the old century passed away were portentous questions of public health. Physicians, editorial writers, and certain enlightened civic leaders had for years lamented Nashville's impure water, inadequate sewage disposal, and smoke. Jere Baxter, president of the Tennessee Central Railroad and competitor of the giant Louisville and Nashville line, blamed the smoke nuisance on the latter. In 1903 the city government sought in vain to enjoin the L&N from using bituminous coal to fire its engines. The polluted air aggravated the suffering from respiratory ailments in Nashville, where 15% of all deaths were attributed to pulmonary tuberculosis. According to the chairman of the Board of Health, this was a rate 50 percent greater than in the nation as a whole.

Numerous families drew drinking water from some 2,000 polluted wells and springs, and the city's own water supply—the Cumberland River—was "wholly bad," declared the Board of Health. The State Bacteriologist in 1909 blamed contaminated water for most cases of typhoid in Nashville. According to survey data, Progressive-era Nashville ranked consistently high among Southern cities in death rates from typhoid, indicating unsanitary conditions, polluted water, or both.

The impure water was due, in part, to infiltration of streams by sewerage. According to Dr. S. S. Crockett, in his valedictory address as president of the Nashville Academy of Medicine in 1905, the problem was the rapid growth of the city.

> "The banks of some of the [Cumberland's] tributary streams are gradually becoming dotted with homes of our citizens and our industrial enterprises, until the revolting possibility is constantly before us of waterborne diseases. . .being served up to us the following morning in our drinking water."

Alongside these nemeses, public officials and private experts condemned tainted food, adulterated drugs, and infected milk sold in Nashville. A city ordinance establishing livestock and food inspection was passed in 1897. After five years, Dr. G. R. White, the meat and livestock inspector, estimated that Nashvillians were still consuming between twenty and thirty thousand pounds of unwholesome meat every year. The local press asserted in 1904 that a "large part of the sickness of the city is due to impure food products." At the Nashville Academy of Medicine, members heard reports from Dr. Lucius P. Brown, State Pure Food and Drug Inspector, on his investigation of unwholesome food in the city.

Other Nashville physicians stressed the significant value of preventive medicine. In a paper read before the Nashville Academy of Medicine in 1905, Dr. John A. Witherspoon urged his colleagues to seek the help of the lay press to educate the public on means of preventing tuberculosis. Eight years later, as president of the American Medical Association, Dr. Witherspoon reiterated his conviction that ". . .today the grandest principle of medicine is to be found in that great modern teaching of prevention."

Concern for infant and child health lay at the heart of preventive medicine and many reforms associated with the "Progressive period" in American history. Dr. S. S.

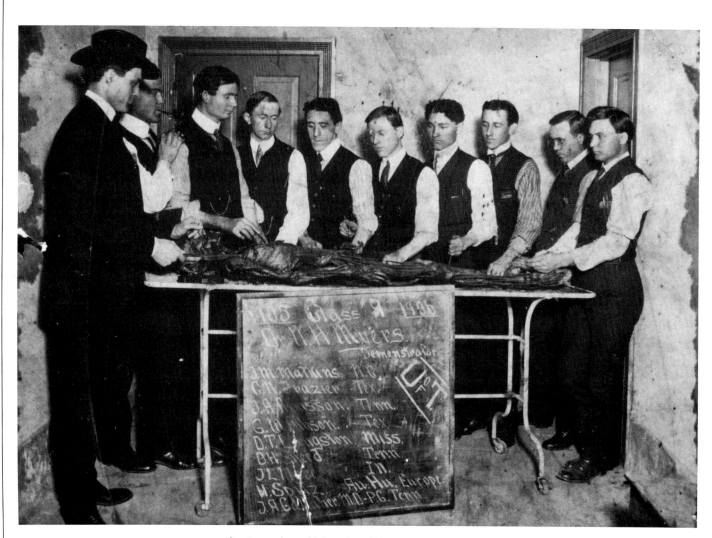

Anatomy class, University of Nashville about 1905

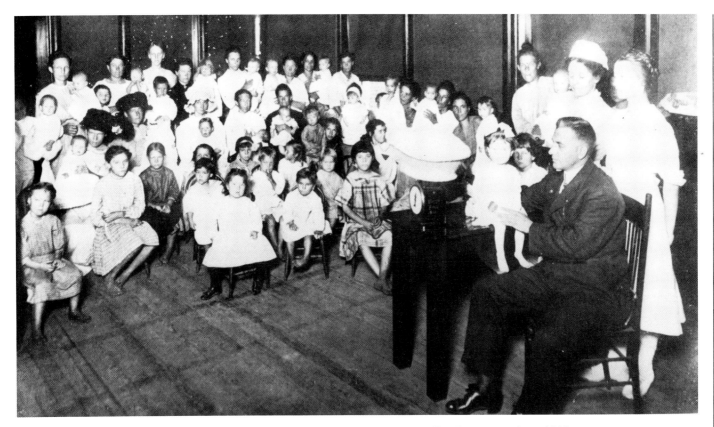

A public health physician examines children at a Nashville dispensary about 1912.
Note the bare feet among several of the youngsters.

Crockett called upon educators to seek the advice of the Nashville Academy of Medicine regarding contagion. A visiting speaker, Dr. Henry Enos Tuley, urged the Academy to work for the betterment of the city's milk supply in the interest of children. The Board of Health set up a department for the care of babies and the prevention of infant death in 1911. Settlement houses, following the example of Jane Adams in Chicago, attacked the high incidence of infant morbidity and mortality in the neighborhoods along the northern and southern tiers of the old city center.

A PURE FOOD AND DRUG LAW

In pursuit of preventive strategies against ill health, the Nashville Academy of Medicine played a key role in the enactment of a state pure food and drug law in 1907. Three one-time Academy presidents—Drs. A. B. Cooke, George H. Price, and S. S. Crockett—worked for its passage. In a welcome address to the convention of the Tennessee State Medical Association in 1913, the Nashville Board of Trade credited an alliance between itself and the city's physicians with passage of a pure milk ordinance and the organization of a commission to study the problem of smoke-polluted air.

The Academy also lent its support to a drive for a smallpox hospital, initiated through the city health officer and the city attorney an ordinance to outlaw spitting on sidewalks, and named the staff physicians at the city's free dispensaries for tuberculosis patients. From time to time the Academy appealed directly to the public to take steps to prevent communicable diseases.

In Dr. Larkin Smith the Board of Health acquired an energetic City Health Officer. Serving from 1898 to 1908, Dr. Smith reorganized the health department and won authority to declare quarantines. The Board possessed other substantial powers: it could order sanitary inspections, direct a scavenger force to abate nuisances, and conduct bacteriological examinations in suspected cases of diphtheria, typhoid fever, malaria, and tuberculosis.

Certain Academy members thought the board was less aggressive than it should be. Dr. John R. Buist, a member of the Board of Health and former Academy president, lamented in 1904 that the City Council often ignored the Board's advice with regard to improving the water, milk, and butter supplies, and tenement regulation; that the health department was understaffed; and that authority over health questions was scattered throughout the municipal bureaucracy.

Dr. W. E. Hibbert, the City Health Officer since 1908, was elected president of the Nashville Academy of Medicine in 1915, a demonstration of the overlapping leadership of the Academy and the Board of Health. Later that year the Academy sought to link itself and its public health agenda to the larger movement of social reform in Nashville. Speaking for the organization, Drs. Hibbert, John Witherspoon, and Olin West called upon the city's commercial, civic, scientific, and professional groups to join

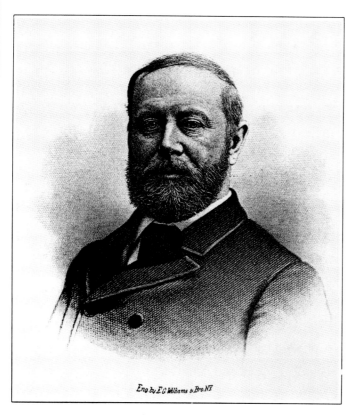

Eng. by E.G. Williams & Bro. NY

Dr. J. R. Buist

with the Academy to form a "Central Health Committee." This panel would study health conditions,

> "uphold public officials in the administration of health laws . . . and serve in whatever manner may become possible for the upbuilding of our community as it can be effected through the protection of health and life from preventable disease and preventable accident."

The preventive aspects of medicine shared the center of the Academy's life and being with clinical, curative, and scientific interests. Each meeting included essays, case reports, and discussions on the treatment of disease. These proceedings regularly appeared in the *Southern Practitioner*, published at Nashville by Dr. Deering J. Roberts, and in the *Journal of the Tennessee Medical Association*.

A number of the Academy's leaders during this period came from the laboratory and the hospital ward. Dr. J. M. King, elected president in 1910, was credited with identifying the first case of pellagra in Nashville. The Academy offered assistance to an intensive study of pellagra conducted at Vanderbilt's medical school in 1915. It also urged the building of a bacteriological laboratory by the city and county, and in 1920 it proposed to finance such a facility with assistance from the Rockefeller Institute. Here was an early proposal for consolidated city-county activity in Nashville that prefigured the joining of those governments more than 50 years later.

THE NATIONAL SCENE

In this same period medical societies sought improved organization of—or at least public peace within—the "factious profession." The continuing development of an organization of doctors in early twentieth century Nashville took place against the backdrop of broad changes in the American Medical Association. At its St. Paul meeting in 1901, the AMA adopted a new constitution that conjoined local societies to it. Thereafter, to belong to the AMA a physician had first to join the local affiliate.

At the beginning of the twentieth century, the chief illnesses that local physicians faced were tuberculosis, typhoid fever, and gastrointestinal diseases of children. It was the era of purgation. A sufferer of any acute illness was usually given a strong emetic, the most popular ones in Tennessee being calomel, castor oil, and epsom salts. Doctors laid great emphasis on "keeping the bowels open." Only then did the physician attempt positive remedies.

Tuberculosis. Even after Robert Koch's identification of the tubercle bacillus in 1882, many people remained skeptical that the disease was contagious. Some insisted that it was hereditary, and thus would sit in a closed room comforting a coughing, dying victim. Physicians could see a 'marked person,' but usually did not mention it to the family, because there was not yet an effective vaccine. The Tennessee doctor tried cod liver oil, hypophosphites, creosote, iodine, cough syrups, opium and sometimes whisky. None did much good. It was not until 1907 that the great clinician William Osler emphasized the value of rest and sunshine.

Typhoid fever. Treatment consisted of rest in bed, and cold baths every two hours if the patient's temperature was above 102 degrees. The doctor prescribed a starvation diet, mainly rice water or barley water, buttermilk, or skimmed milk. Egg albumin in lemonade was also acceptable, and doubtless more palatable.

Dr. J. T. Moore, Sr. (University of Tennessee School of Medicine, Nashville, 1904) wrote of trying a supposed intestinal antiseptic drug, and lost two little girls to the disease. "From that day to this, I have never used a new drug until it has been thoroughly tested and recommended by our best authorities," he recalled nearly fifty years after his young patients' deaths.

Children's diseases. Gastrointestinal infections were likewise treated first by purgation, then a starvation diet. With the discovery of the diphtheria antitoxin by Emil Berhing in 1892, doctors were handed a powerful weapon. With its administration "and intubation in laryngeal cases, it was very unusual to have a fatal case," Dr. Moore observed.

Tennessee parents still relied on their own home remedies and therapies for treating children, just as their grandmothers had done on the frontier. Coal oil was given for croup. Certain old persons were deemed to have a special insight into treating children and would be allowed to blow into a baby's mouth to cure the "thrash." All little ones were destined to have mumps, measles, and chicken pox, in which cases the doctor's best help was imparting information and understanding to worried parents.

The first fruits of modern pharmacology in medicine were being realized in Tennessee. For example, malaria responded to quinine, and for anemia, the doctor prescribed iron quinine and strychnine in tonic doses. Still a century ago, a doctor had to contend with ignorance on the part of many patients and faith doctors, quacks, and even witchery. It required state power before these last were driven from the field, although "cancer doctors" with empty promises preyed on desperate people far into the twentieth century.

Subsequently the AMA created a model constitution for state societies that fixed a like condition: no member of the national association unless also a member of the state body of doctors.

Dr. Joseph N. McCormick, a resourceful and energetic organizer, traveled extensively throughout the nation between 1903 and 1911, crusading for the adoption of the model state constitution and otherwise assisting state societies to unify and strengthen themselves. As a result, membership in physicians' organizations at all levels grew dramatically. The Tennessee State Medical Association, for example, swelled from 400 to 1,200 following its reorganization in 1902.

The greater number of physicians enrolled in societies multiplied their potential political strength, and the AMA urged state bodies to create committees to review all health bills introduced in legislatures. Its own Committee on Medical Legislation drafted model medical practice and vital statistics statutes, urged enforcement of the national Pure Food and Drug Act, and cited Tennessee's law on that subject as among the best, one that other states might imitate.

The AMA further strengthened its authority as it organized bureaus and councils to examine a broad spectrum of issues. These bodies carried on extensive educational and public relations work, frequently in association with state public health agencies and local chapters of national civic organizations. In 1914 the AMA Council on Health and Public Instruction outlined several public policy goals. To the medical practice acts, vital statistics laws, and pure food and drug statutes, it added new water quality and sewerage disposal standards, called for state sanitary surveys, and urged the expansion of local health department activities in coordination with state health boards. Promotion of laws to reduce industrial disease and to provide for milk inspection and medical inspection of schools concluded the list. During the Progressive era, the AMA largely achieved this ambitious agenda by reinforcing and expanding the alliance with the law that

sanitarians had achieved in Nashville and other localities during the late nineteenth century.

In Nashville some changes came harder than others. When the Nashville Academy of Medicine admitted a woman member in 1901, "Medicus," writing in the *Nashville Banner*, ascribed the action to a "temporary obfuscation of the ethico-intellectual faculties" of his colleagues. "This proud and social centre of the South," he feared, might "evolve a shrieking Anna Dickinson, a howling Ellen Lease, and a smashing Carrie Nation."

At the beginning of the new century, membership of the medical academy stood at 85. A new constitution and by-laws adopted in 1903 (revising those of 1897) opened membership to "every legally registered physician residing and practicing in Davidson County, who is of good moral and professional standing and who does not practice or claim to practice sectarian medicine." This standard reflected the AMA's position: beginning in 1903 its local affiliates were allowed to admit all physicians not supporting an exclusive system.

Although the American Institute of Homeopathy resisted the AMA's overtures, most homeopathic physicians agreed with the view that basic biomedical sciences were necessary preparations for all students. As the scientific bases of the two traditions converged, regular physicians put aside their enmity. Dr. Lucius E. Burch, president of the Nashville Academy of Medicine in 1905-06, told a graduating class at Vanderbilt medical school:

> "... It is your purpose to relieve suffering and to bring people to health and happiness; and that after you have diagnosed the case, whatever remedy seems best to you should be applied without considering for a moment sect or creed. You will often be consulted as to the value of certain patent medicines, homeopathic remedies, Christian science, and maybe osteopathy; and if you find it advisable to use any of these treatments, do so without hesitation."

As part of its development and expansion, the Nashville Academy of Medicine concluded an arrangement with Carnegie Library to care for its books and journals. For several years members met in the library, then moved sessions next door to Tulane Hotel, fronting on Church Street. Both buildings stood adjacent to the densest concentration of physicians' offices in the city.

With this proximity to the Capitol, Nashville doctors became the lobbying arm of organized medicine in Tennessee. In 1921-22, three of the five members of the state medical association's committee on public policy and legislation resided in Nashville. The leadership of the Academy and the state society interpenetrated and overlapped. Of the presidents of the State Association between 1900 and 1921, six were Nashvillians. When the state group started its *Journal* in 1908, the publications committee comprised three one-time Academy presidents.

In efforts to influence public policy, the medical profession declared that the public's interest was its interest, just as it had done in the public health campaigns of the late nineteenth century. Those efforts to encourage the cleansing of the city required popular acceptance of the connection between filth and disease. Expressed another way, reform in public health required participation by people and judgment from them.

To lead that movement physicians urged the creation of state and local health boards. Naturally they were the logical appointees, and thus in place to guide whatever initiatives governments undertook.

At the same time, as scientific medicine promised therapeutic advances, it placed the doctor beyond the reach of public judgment. Exhorted by physicians not to spit on the sidewalks, Nashvillians might assume responsibility for controlling tuberculosis. But only physicians trained in laboratory methods could evaluate the latest pronouncements from Koch's institute. As they declared scientific training to be the mark of a physician, they gathered greater authority to themselves than their generation's predecessors had ever enjoyed.

REFORMING MEDICAL EDUCATION

For half a century organized medicine had declared that the only true physician was the well-educated one, but doctors had failed to define and then achieve control over requirements in medical colleges. Throughout the last quarter of the nineteenth century, national and regional associations of medical educators urged medical schools to stiffen their admissions requirements and make more rigorous their curricula. By 1900 these proposals generally included a four-year, postgraduate course of study centered in laboratories and in bedside teaching at a hospital connected with the medical school. Students' training would be divided between preclinical (first and second) years and clinical (third and fourth) years. As seen in the proceedings of the Nashville and Tennessee medical societies, local leaders had long called for fewer, better-trained physicians. Finally, in the state and in the nation, these goals were accomplished within a generation, roughly the period from the spread of licensing statutes to the establishment of minimum standards for medical schools, all of it set into law by state legislatures. In Tennessee the first licensing law had been enacted in 1889. The requirements in the University of Tennessee medical school were made the minimum standard for other medical schools in 1919.

The licensing law set created a state board of medical examiners that recognized homeopaths and eclectics as well as "allopaths," that is doctors who did not advocate or adhere to a system. For twelve years the board actually applied more stringent standards for licensure, and the General Assembly gave it authority to refuse to recognized diplomas form colleges not "in good standing." In 1892 it began requiring that candidates for licensure submit to a written as well as an oral examination and present evidence of a pre-medical education. The Board deemed these additional requirements necessary because standards in Tennessee' medical schools were generally considered low. In 1900 the secretary of the medical examiners board testified before the legislative committee of the state medical society. His words could have described the state of educating doctors a hundred years earlier:

> "Some individuals have procured diplomas by enrolling at colleges without attending the lectures. . . . More than one college has received students and granted them a diploma upon examination without requiring attendance upon lectures."

In 1901 the state medical association captured control over the board by successful lobbying for repeal of the 1889 act. The new law gave regular physicians—those who did not adhere to or advocate a system—four of the six seats on a newly-constituted licensing board. (Omission of the term "allopathic" from the statute, formerly used to describe regular or non-sectarian doctors, was itself a triumph from the state medical association's point of view.)

Besides giving regular physicians a two-thirds majority on the new board, the 1901 law required that anyone seeking a license to practice medicine in Tennessee must pass an examination that the Board administered. A diploma, by itself, was now no longer a sufficient condition for licensure. The Board was further empowered to revoke licenses of physicians found guilty of "unprofessional or dishonorable conduct." The act defined this to mean performing or procuring criminal abortion; accepting fees to cure incurable disease; betraying professional secrets; false advertising, including specifically that related to female disorders; moral turpitude; and intemperance or drug addiction. Finally the act curtailed the practices of itinerant physicians or vendors of drugs and nostrums.

The licensing of doctors was made still more restrictive in 1915 when the General Assembly created the State Board of Preliminary Examinations. This law, unanimously endorsed by the Nashville Academy of Medicine, required that prior to taking the licensing examination an applicant must obtain certification from the preliminary examinations board that he or she was a high school graduate as well as a diplomate in medicine. This new statute also provided that by 1919 the standards of all medical colleges in the state must at least equal those of the medical department of the University of Tennessee.

Although state power gave the new standards in medical education force and effect, in the Progressive era the American Medical Association defined, then lobbied for the establishment of those standards on a lasting, national basis. In 1906 the AMA's Committee on Medical Education divided the medical schools of the country into four classes according the percentage of their graduates failing state licensing examinations. That fall it conducted its first inspection of medical schools, using a ten-point standard to test the capacity of each institution to offer an acceptable education. Colleges that failed to obtain a rating of 70 would not be recognized by the AMA, and it urged that states also deny them recognition.

Thus, even before the 1910 study of American medical education by Abraham Flexner and the Carnegie Foundation, the medical profession began to set educational standards and win the underpinning of state power for them. Flexner's survey nonetheless played a role in the institutional transformation of Progressive-era medicine in Nashville, as elsewhere.

THE FLEXNER REPORT

Flexner found no medical school in that city that fully met his and his sponsor's ideal—a full-time faculty, adequate pre-clinical preparation by students, a four-year course divided between basic sciences and clinical experience, and an internship. He commended recent improvements at the Universities of Nashville and Tennessee Medical Department, but criticized its laboratory, dissecting room, and part-time faculty. Vanderbilt University's medical school also lacked a single full-time instructor; Flexner went on to describe its dissecting room as "foul" and its clinical offerings as inadequate. Meharry Medical College received high marks; indeed, Flexner recommended that, of the seven medical schools for blacks in the United States, only Meharry and that of Howard University be aided by philanthropists.

Flexner's recommendation that the University of Tennessee abandon its effort to teach medicine was carried out promptly. The department that it had operated jointly with the University of Nashville since 1909 was discontinued in 1911, the faculty combining with Vanderbilt. The closing of its medical school effectively marked the end of the venerable University of Nashville, which Flexner described as "a university in name only."

With certain fundamental changes, which he specified in detail, Flexner believed that Vanderbilt could be well-situated to serve as Tennessee's medical school. Northern philanthropy followed his counsel. William K. Vanderbilt and the Education Board of New York each gave the

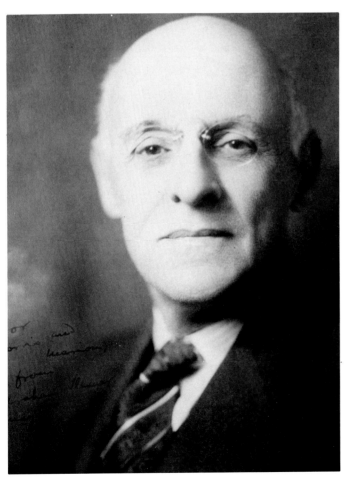

Dr. Abraham Flexner

Vanderbilt medical school $150,000 in 1911. Andrew Carnegie contributed one million dollars two years later. The General Education Board of the Rockefeller Foundation, viewing the institution as potentially a model for the South, contributed four million in 1919, conditioned upon the adoption the full-time clinical faculty rule that the Board required of its beneficiaries.

Its students barred from the City Hospital, Meharry Medical College attained the standard of bedside teaching in medicine by sending upperclassmen to Mercy Hospital, built and owned by Dr. Robert Fulton Boyd (Meharry, M.D., 1882, D.D.S., 1887) In 1910 the college opened its own uncompleted George W. Hubbard Hospital. "No Eastern capital used," it proudly told the press. However, Andrew Carnegie gave $10,000 to help finish the facility, which had been commended by Abraham Flexner. In 1919 Carnegie gave another $150,000, as did the General Education Board.

Meharry had been founded by Methodist missionaries in 1876, in response to the high rates of sickness and untimely death among blacks in the Reconstruction South. The enterprise soon won support from civic leaders and other authorities, who argued that the presence of disease-ridden blacks imperiled whites living around and among them. As the twentieth century dawned, blacks were, in the minds of many white Nashvillians, the proximate cause of much illness in the city. Their supposed congenital disposition, especially to tuberculosis, encouraged state laws and local ordinances crafted to confine blacks to their own precincts. In Nashville restrictive covenants fixed boundaries to black neighborhoods, usually the sections of town with the worst housing, poorest drainage, and industrial smoke and waste. The rigid segregation of the era was fostered in part by fear of blacks as a health menace, a fear not without a rational basis. Morbidity and mortality in the city's Negro neighborhoods were frequently 50% greater than in white areas of town.

Given these differentially high rates of illness and untimely death among their patients, black physicians greatly needed the exchange of information available from association with fellow doctors. Like their white colleagues, they sought the fraternity, fellowship, and recognition that medical society membership offered. Finally, just as the AMA asserted its members claims of competence, black doctors believed that, by organizing, they could raise public confidence in their ability and authority.

In 1880, three years after he became Meharry's first graduate, Dr. James Monroe Jamison and others among the eighteen black physicians in the state, founded the Tennessee "Colored Medical Association." No further activity of this society is known; it was not mentioned in Dr. Myles V. Link's *Medical and Surgical Observer*, the first black medical journal in the United States, published at Jackson, Tennessee from 1892 to 1894.

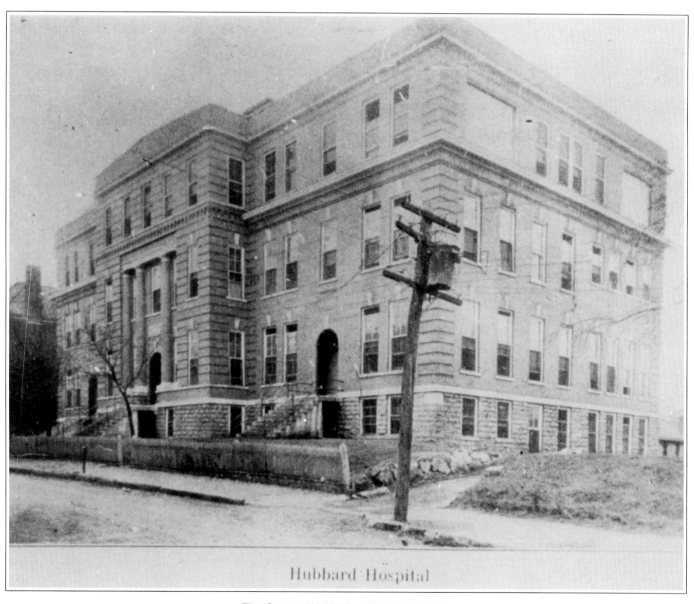

The George W. Hubbard Hospital, 1910

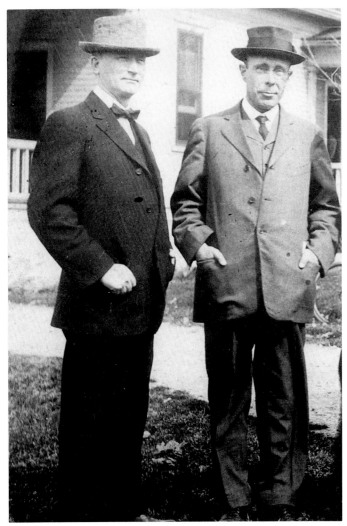
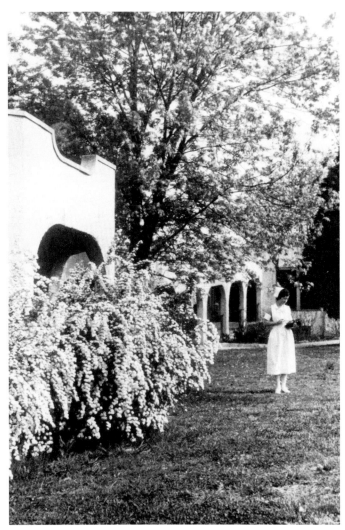

Above, left: Dr. Edward A. Sutherland, left, and Dr. Percy T. Magan were among the founders of the Madison Rural Sanitarium, which stressed natural remedies such as sunshine, exercise, and nutritious diets low in sugar and fat. By the 1930's the Madison Rural Sanitarium, as it was then called, grew to eight hundred acres, one hundred rooms, state of the art medical equipment, and fourteen physicians on staff. This institution was the forerunner of today's Tennessee Christian Medical Center. **Above, right:** The sanitarium about 1940. The nurse is ringing a tone box announcing a meal time.

BLACK PHYSICIANS ORGANIZE

Black practitioners, including surgeons, dentists, and pharmacists, established the National Medical Association at the Cotton States Exposition in Atlanta in 1895. During the next eight years, three NMA presidents—Robert Fulton Boyd, Henry T. Noel, and Ferdinand A. Stewart—came from Nashville. Three times during its early years (in 1897, 1903, and 1913) the NMA held its annual convention in the city.

Three months before the 1903 meeting, black practitioners of Nashville organized in the Medico-Chirurgical Society, invited colleagues across Tennessee to meet with them to form a state group. On August 20, thirty-four physicians, dentists, and pharmacists convened in the Capitol and set up the Negro Medical Congress of Tennessee. Its purposes, described in its constitution, were to "discuss, advised, and adopt the best means to disseminate hygienic measures for our people and for mutual help for our fellow laborers." By 1915 this organization was known by its permanent name, the Volunteer State Medical Association.

Whether the Nashville Society of Colored Physicians, also meeting in 1903, was the same as the Medico-Chirurgical Society is unknown. The black medical profession was as rife with factions and jealousies as its white counterpart; however, black doctors, like other physicians of the era, may simply have reorganized periodically under various names. In 1907 they met as the Nashville Academy of Medicine, Dentistry, and Pharmacy before taking the name Rock City Academy of Medicine and Surgery, an allusion to Nashville's foundation of Ordovician limestone and a popular old nickname of the city.

Nashville's black doctors believed that hygienic conditions in Negro neighborhoods followed from degraded political and social conditions there. They insisted that improvements in Negro health required educational and preventive approaches. Having little influence over the regulatory or prescriptive power of the state against such threats as impure food, tenement housing, drugs, and vice, black practitioners could only warn their patients to care for their own conditions of health by asserting a measure of control over their lives and neighborhoods. Here was one of the ambiguous outcomes of the rigid segregation of the period: an increase in self-sufficiency, self-identity, and self-assertion among black Nashvillians.

The Rock City Academy of Medicine sponsored an annual health week that included a public meeting. At this event in 1910 Academy members lectured on hookworm, pellagra, tuberculosis, the fly-borne diseases, and "the duty of the Negro to the profession." Mayor Hilary Howse and City Health Officer W. E. Hibbett also addressed the audience. According to Dr. Arthur M. Townsend (Meharry Class of 1902), echoes from the meeting "reverberated through the valleys of negligence and carelessness in Nashville...Herein lies one of our greatest missions as an organization—to teach the people how to prevent disease."

Dr. Townsend, who served as the Rock City Academy's president from 1906 to 1908, declared a further objective, the achievement of recognition and authority for Negro physicians. Lamenting blacks' inclination to doubt the ability of a practitioner of their own race, he testified in articles and speeches that his colleagues were "able to do anything in medicine and surgery so far as research has been able to find." He saw the success of the black physician as literally a vital issue in the community:

> "Where our people carry out the principles of employing Negro doctors, the statistics as filed in the office of the health department of the city show that mortality in such communities is far less than where other conditions obtain."

Beginning in June, 1910 Nashville's black medical society conducted annual summer clinics at Meharry to treat sufferers who could not afford to pay. As a result, Dr. Townsend told his colleagues, these charity patients would not have to go to "some other institution, where under the garb of nice treatment and free service, they take advantage of our people for experimental purposes."

Dr. Townsend credited the Academy with being the model for other black civic and professional organizations. Its authority, he wrote, was such that "any regulation we may deem best to adopt pertaining to the profession is willingly accepted as authority by the people," and he noted that the group was "the moving spirit in the State Association, and regarded as such." Leaders among black physicians associated themselves with the city health department's war against tuberculosis, and there was an overlapping leadership between the Rock City Academy and the Anti-Tuberculosis League, formed in 1906 with Dr. Robert Fulton Boyd as president. In time, after his death, Nashville's organization of black physicians was named for Dr. Boyd.

Creation by black people of institutions—including an organized medical profession—to serve themselves was part of their resistance to the era's pervasive and virulent segregation. In its new constitution and by-laws of 1913, the Nashville Academy of Medicine for the first time inserted race among the criteria for membership eligibility, providing that "every legally registered white physician" might belong.

Along with this signature of the times, the new organic document incorporated the locutions of Progressivism. The statement of "Purposes of the Society" suggests a profession shedding the anxieties that had beset it only a few years before. Here was a called for "intelligent unity and harmony" to "elevate and make effective the opinions of the profession in all scientific, legislative, public health, material, and social affairs." The goal was "to receive that respect and support within its own ranks, and from the community, to which its honorable history and great achievements entitle it."

One of its achievements was the economic advancement of the sodality, the purpose of the first Nashville medical society almost a century before. When the Academy served as host to the Southern Medical Association's annual convention in 1910, its president praised the local group for its "great economic value" to physicians in Nashville. No fee schedule from this period has come to light; such schedules made public or discovered by the press in other localities sometimes led to press attacks on the "medical trust." The existence of such a schedule is implied in a 1908 editorial in the *Nashville Journal of Medicine and Surgery*. According to editor Charles S. Briggs:

> The fee bill is a necessity for it establishes a standard of charges that regulates fees to some extent and puts a legal valuation upon medical services and gives the patient some idea of what he may be expected to pay.

He added:

> That we as professional men are not better paid is a fault within ourselves. We do not uphold each other and are too prone to be lax in our collections and to estimate our services at too small a figure.... Physicians the world over are proverbially deficient in business acumen and as a consequence the medical profession is the poorest paid profession in the world.

Such exhortation, and a practical chart of minimum charges may have played their role in raising physicians' incomes. But the decisive reason was a decrease in competition. The 1920 census showed 186 physicians and surgeons in Nashville, whose population was 118,342. This was only nineteen more doctors than the 267 who, in 1900, had served 80,865 residents. To put the point in a different way, Nashville's population had grown by 46.5% over 20 years' time, but its supply of physicians by just 7.1% This consequence of steepening standards in education and licensure, writ large throughout the nation, helped to achieve the rise in public respect for physicians that the leadership of organized medicine in Nashville had long sought.

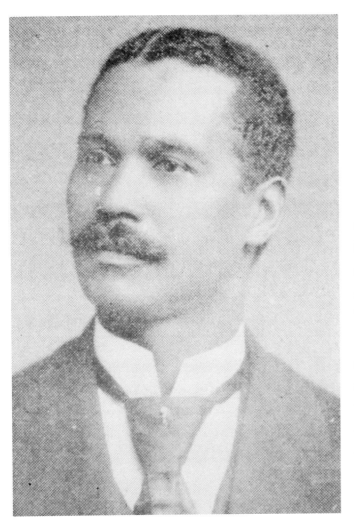

Dr. Robert Fulton Boyd

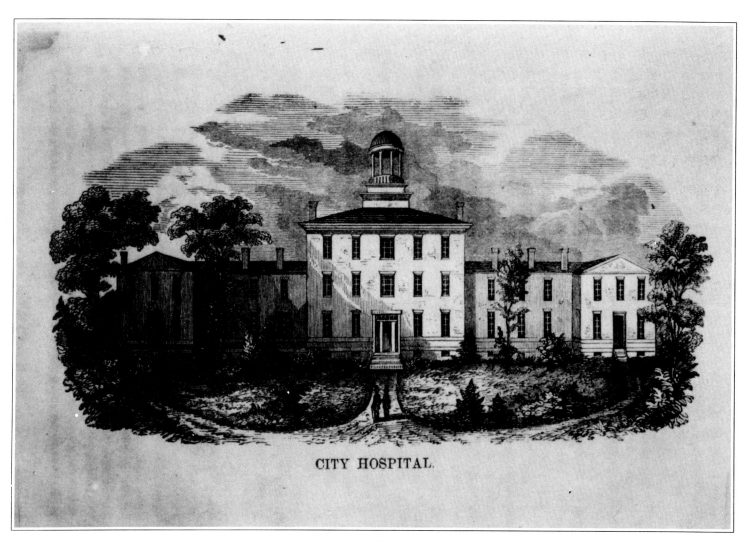

CITY HOSPITAL.

The first City Hospital

Chapter Six

THE GREAT AGE OF HOSPITAL BUILDING

---

*I*n the half-century from 1870 to 1920, Nashville saw the rise of a large civic institution, the hospital. Such places, to be sure, had predecessors in former days. In 1847 Dorothea Dix addressed the Tennessee General Assembly, eloquently lamenting the deplorable conditions at the insane asylum, built in 1833 near present-day Eighth and Broad. In 1848 lawmakers provided funds for a new 250-bed facility on Murfreesboro Road, and it received its first patients in the winter of 1852. The Sisters of Charity of Nazareth opened St. John's Hospital at Gay Street and present-day Sixth Avenue, North, in the late 1840s, the first of several orders of Catholic women whose work marks the hospital history of the city.

Hospitals had from their beginning been enterprises founded and run by charitable groups. Nashville in time received such boons from the Baptists, the Catholics, the Methodists, Seventh Day Adventists, and others. By the early twentieth century, medical schools became a second progenitor of hospitals, as bedside teaching became a requirement for the training of doctors. Not coincidentally, these same years saw the winnowing out of the city's medical schools. Two—Meharry and Vanderbilt—survived the wave of reform begun by the A.M.A. and culminating in the Flexner Report. Small proprietory schools could not meet the new standards, of which an emphasis on bedside teaching was key.

VANDERBILT AND THE UNIVERSITY OF TENNESSEE

The combined medical department of Vanderbilt and the University of Nashville Vanderbilt, whose origin is discussed in the sidebar beginning on page 42, opened a hospital in 1875. Catalogues promised that students would have "abundant clinical material" drawn from the State Penitentiary and St. Vincent's Hospital, a facility opened by the University of Nashville before the war.

The highly competitive nature of medical practice followed into medical education when Drs. Duncan Eve and W. Frank Glenn formed Nashville Medical College in the summer of 1876. They drew from—or at least had permission to use the names of—noted faculty members of the Vanderbilt and University of Nashville medical department. The

Below and opposite: Government's growing role in medicine was visible in charitable institutions, including hospitals.

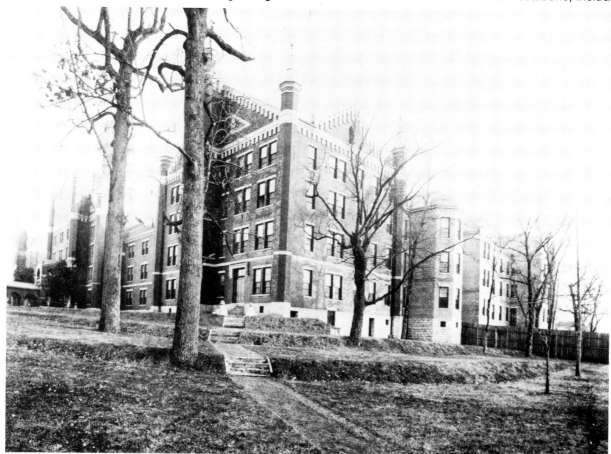

State Insane
Asylum,
early 1890s

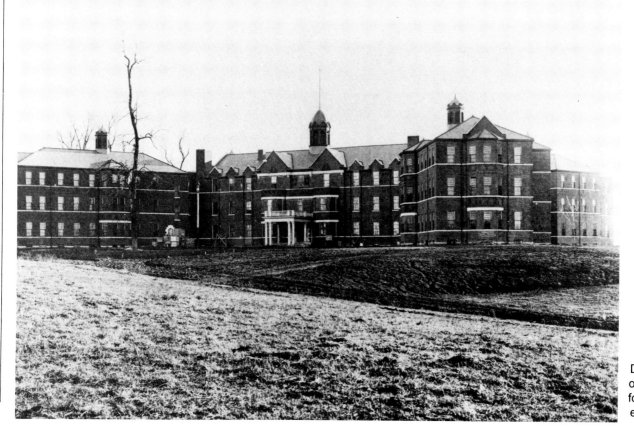

Insane
Department
of the Home
for the Poor,
early 1890s

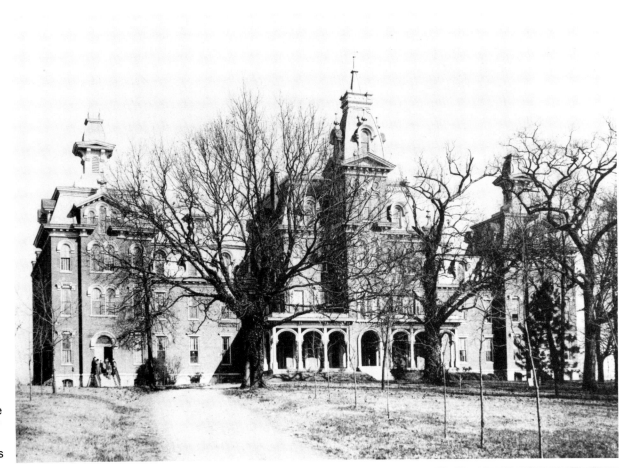

Tennessee
School for
the Blind,
early 1890s

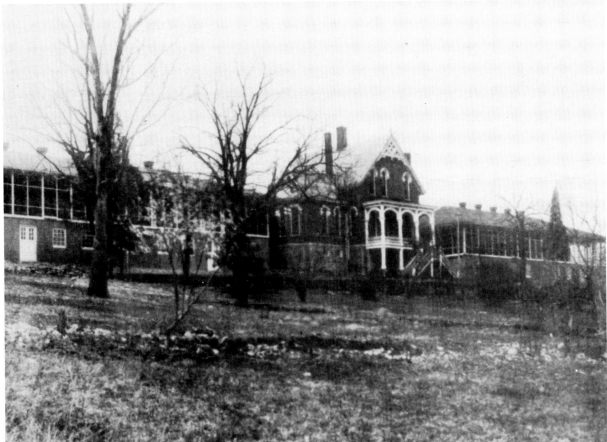

Nashville
and
Davidson
County's
tuberculosis
hospital, at
the time of its
opening
in1912

school was adopted by the University of Tennessee as its medical department in 1879 and the next year, it founded a hospital on Broad Street, between present-day Sixth and Seventh Avenues.

When the partnership between the University of Nashville dissolved, in 1895 Vanderbilt opened its own medical campus at Fifth Avenue, South, and Elm Street, on old College Hill in South Nashville. Down the street at Second and Elm, the University of Nashville built a new medical building. Here in 1909 the University of Tennessee's Nashville Medical College and the University of Nashville merged to train doctors. The former's old building on Broad became a teaching facility, Tennessee Hospital.

Vanderbilt also erected a new medical school building at Fifth Avenue, South, and Elm Street. For a time it appeared that this old section of town would become its second major hospital campus, along with the Murphy suburb: near the medical schools' facilities the Methodist Church began building Galloway Memorial Hospital (named for a bishop of the church) in 1912. By 1919 it was still not completed, and the property was deeded to Vanderbilt. That same year Chancellor James H. Kirkland won a grant of four million dollars from the Rockefeller Foundation, conditioned on the promise that the University would go to the full-time plan for faculty and adopt other recommendations put forward in the Flexner report. Vanderbilt chose to begin from the ground up, and at a different place, its west campus. There between 1921 and 1925 an entirely new medical school and hospital rose.

HUBBARD HOSPITAL

Meharry's teaching hospital was founded out of two deep social forces. One was the plight of sick people among Nashville's black population. In every census and public health report, blacks suffered greater rates of morbidity and untimely mortality than whites. Proportionately more black infants than white infants succumbed to diseases of the very young. Communicable diseases like tuberculosis and diphtheria cut wider swaths through the black neighborhoods of the city than through its white sections.

The rising standards in medical education also drove the development of a hospital at Meharry Medical College. Dr. Robert Fulton Boyd's infirmary served as a limited teaching facilities throughout the 1890s, but it was small, its equipment limited, and surgery was a rare event. Meharry had to offer bedside teaching and practice, the observation and experience of disease, not merely a textbook and lectures.

Meharry's president, Dr. George W. Hubbard, unwittingly set in motion events leading to the building of the hospital that would one day be named for him. Attending a conference on standards and curricula in Chicago in 1899, he sought to recruit to his faculty Dr. Daniel Hale Williams, whom one fervent admirer called the "bright and morning star in the firmament of Negro surgery." Williams had won the sobriquet in 1893 when he performed a suture of the pericardium to repair a knife wound, an operation that some have called the first successful heart surgery in history.

Dr. Williams agreed to hold some surgical clinics at Meharry and in 1899 he did four successful operations in the cramped rooms of the Boyd infirmary. Nonetheless, he was not impressed with the facility. Before he left Nashville, he expressed candidly to Dr. Hubbard the need for a hospital experience for Meharry students. If Nashville's City Hospital would not admit blacks to study or work there, there was only one solution: they must build their own hospital that would include a training program for nurses.

The Chicago surgeon returned to Nashville the following year to exhort local leaders to rent a house, furnish it modestly, gather the best physicians available—and open the doors. In September, 1900, Mercy Hospital began serving the community in a building that Dr. Boyd had purchased. Dr. Williams came back from time to time to conduct surgical clinics there.

The building grew from twelve to three dozen beds, yet

it remained crowded and Meharry did not own it. In the meantime, other Meharry faculty who resented the preference given this institution by the college started competing facilities and demanded a portion of the college's budget that subsidized Mercy.

Once again Dr. Boyd seized the initiative and proposed that Meharry now build the real hospital that Dr. Williams had envisioned might grow from a modest start. The fundraising effort proved hard, but with major support from Andrew Carnegie, in 1916 Hubbard Hospital opened its doors on the south Nashville campus. Besides serving as the teaching hospital of the medical school, it continued the nursing education program that had commenced at Mercy, and by the mid-1930s more than 200 women had graduated in nursing at Hubbard Hospital and were established in practice in nearly every state in the Union.

A HOSPITAL FOR THE PUBLIC

Memoirs of the day record the life of temptation and dissolution that many young people in Gilded Age Nashville faced. In the 1880s and 1890s the city was brought to its knees by the sermons of evangelist Sam Jones, who charged its leading men with neglecting a host of problems. While his plea was for redemption from sin, he unleashed a torrent of social concern. At the same time the voters sent to the Mayor's office in 1872 Republican Thomas Kercheval, and they reelected him for twelve two-year terms.

During the Kercheval years, the city council appropriated money to build a public hospital, which had been authorized in 1879 but never funded. In April, 1890, the institution opened its doors on Rolling Mill Hill, so called because it was the site of milling plants in an earlier day

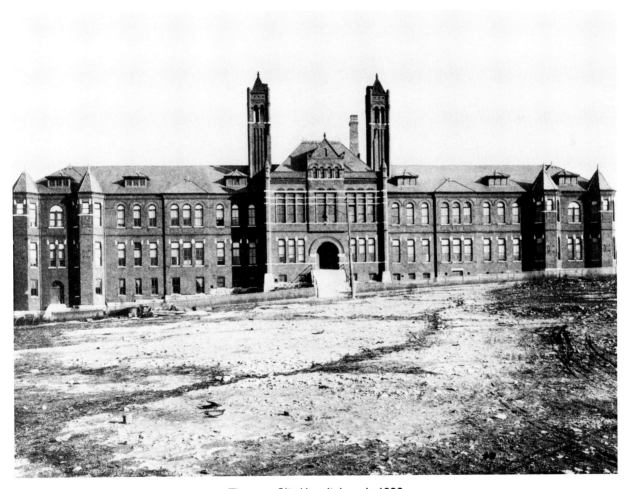

The new City Hospital, early 1890s

when Nashville turned corn from the hinterlands into flour. Officially called City Hospital at first, it eventually became known as General. The consulting staff included Drs. Duncan and Paul F. Eve, Jr., in surgery; Drs. J. H. Cain and J. H. Blanks, in medicine; Dr. William D. Haggard in gynecology and pediatrics; and Dr. J. G. Sinclair, in diseases of the eye, ear, nose, and throat. Each served on the faculty of the University of Tennessee, and now its students had new opportunity for clinical instruction.

Dr. Charles Brower, a graduate of the University of Nashville,

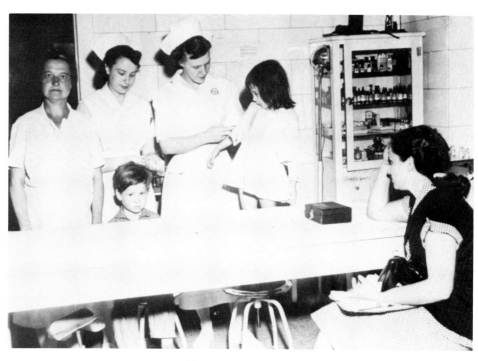

The outpatient clinic

served as the first superintendent of the 60-bed, four-ward institution. Two years after taking charge, he observed that mortality statistics of patients were "not surpassed by any [hospital] in the United States." Patient records reveal gender and color, occupation, and nativity and show that the hospital took in chambermaids and gamblers, midwives and prostitutes, saddlers, soap makers, saloon keepers, and teamsters.

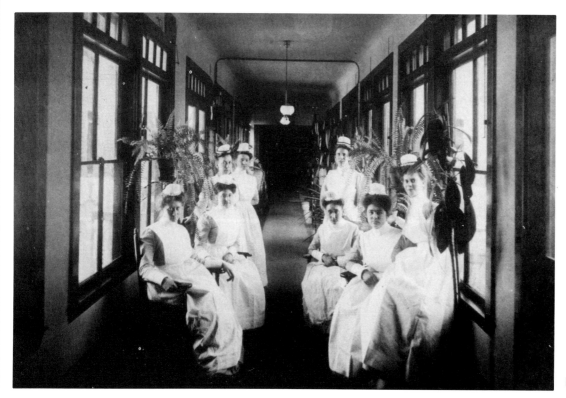

Part of the nursing staff

In 1892 a school of nursing opened at City Hospital, only the second one in the South. Miss Charlotte E. Perkins, alumna of the Pennsylvania Hospital Training School, directed the school, which continued until 1970. By the end of the decade City Hospital was staffed by Dr. Brower and seven nurses.

Until 1921 a single physician continued to treat all the charity patients who came through the doors of the institution, although six years earlier a wing had been added to accommodate private patients. Faculty members and students from Vanderbilt and the University of Tennessee (until it relocated) also used its wards for teaching.

In 1921 the hospital underwent a thorough renovation. The numbers of nurses in training and supervising nurses were increased. Kitchens, pharmacy, and childrens ward were improved, and the board of hospital commissioners promised a new home for nurses and new operating rooms. In 1932 a new wing increased the bed capacity to 260. Chaired by Dr. Rufus E. Fort, the board comprised four physicians and three lay civic leaders.

The Davidson County Asylum and Poor House began in 1893 as a facility for people suffering mental affliction and a home for persons chronically ill who could not support and care for themselves. A three-story structure, it comprised a central administration building and two patient wings and was surrounded by 650 acres, with a dairy, cannery, laundry, and farm buildings. The institution had been authorized by the county court—the lawmaking body of Davidson County—in 1892 to replace the

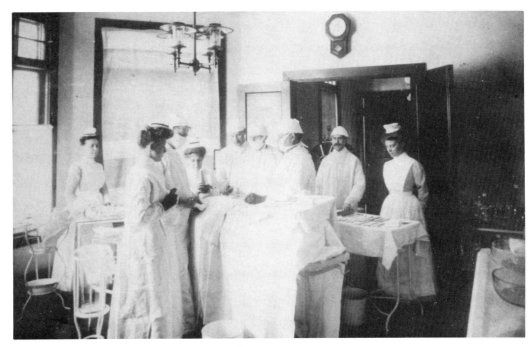

Surgery team

Asylum for the Poor and Insane operating on Gallatin Road since 1874. When the new facility opened on December 7, 1893, 200 paupers and 95 insane persons were moved on that day, and none missed a meal.

In 1917 two new wings were added to the original structure, known as the Core Addition for Dr. W. W. Core, superintendent from 1900 to 1936. Dr. Core's assistant at the time was Dr. John J. Lentz, later director of public health for Davidson County and for the Metropolitan Government. Dr. Core was succeeded by Dr. Henry B. Brackin, Sr.

THE INFIRMARY MOVEMENT

For persons who could afford the charges, private infirmaries offered eminent physicians' personal attention and total discretion. The Nashville Infirmary, flourishing in 1876, charged $8-14 a week for private rooms. The advertisements for the Douglas Infirmary, Dr. Richard Douglas, proprietor, appeared in the newspapers and city directories of the day. Drs. Richard Barr, Lucius Burch, and William T. Briggs operated private clinics like these well into the twentieth century. In a sense, they continued and built upon the older tradition of the physician in the free market. Here well-to-do families could shield their members from notoriety. Such proprietors lived by public favor and referrals, their standing among colleagues and in the community depending on the family backgrounds of the people they treated. Paul Starr has called them "medical courtiers."

These infirmaries captured patients seeking convalescence, which physicians could offer with confidence. But other changes—in society and in medicine—transformed hospitals into entirely new kinds of institutions and brought them new patrons and sponsors.

Advances in surgery made it sensible for hospitals to serve recuperating patients, who required not merely pallative but active care, such as nurses could provide. Thus hospitals gave rise to nurse training schools. Hubbard Hospital undertook this role, as did St. Thomas, Baptist, and Vanderbilt. Out of these grew schools of nursing. Only in the hospital could physicians practice asepsis, their great weapon against post-operative infection.

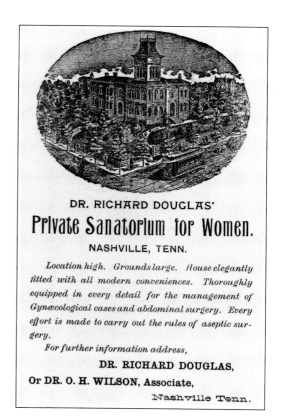

DR. RICHARD DOUGLAS'
Private Sanatorium for Women.
NASHVILLE, TENN.

Location high. Grounds large. House elegantly fitted with all modern conveniences. Thoroughly equipped in every detail for the management of Gynæcological cases and abdominal surgery. Every effort is made to carry out the rules of aseptic surgery.

For further information address,

DR. RICHARD DOUGLAS,
Or DR. O. H. WILSON, Associate,

Nashville Tenn.

Dr. Richard Douglas' Private Sanatorium catered to the needs of affluent Nashville women.

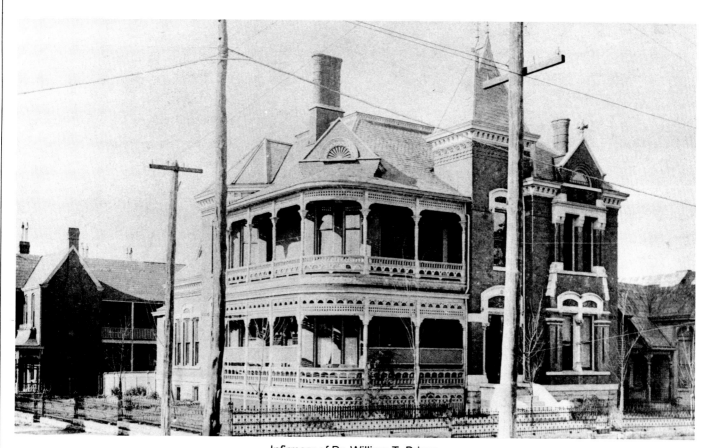

Infirmary of Dr. William T. Briggs

Hospital appointments became valuable to other specialists in the years at the hinge of the centuries. Meeting patients in that setting the doctor could concentrate his time. Hospitals, especially public hospitals, coincided with important demographic and social changes in Nashville and other cities. As jobs in factories and on railroads and in the banking and insurance companies drew people to Nashville, they in many cases became more strained by misfortune, like illness.

St. Thomas Hospital

The Catholic Church experienced a resurgence of communicants in Nashville when the city received a great stream of Irish immigrants before the war. By 1880 one in every eight Nashvillians had been born in Ireland or was first generation Irish-American. In the late years of the century their mother church began one of Nashville's great hospitals.

The Daughters of Charity were the spiritual heirs of St. Vincent de Paul and Saint Louise de Marilac, who founded a community of religious women in Paris in 1633. The two organized and trained young women to do charitable work, such as providing food and other necessities, among poor people of the city. The Daughters' mission grew; they taught children, cared for sick in hospitals and soldiers from battlefields. The order started orphanages, homes for old people, private halls for unwed mothers, hostels for beggars—their charity encompassed the stages of man.

Elizabeth Ann Seton brought their work to the United States. She established the Daughters in Emmitsburg, Maryland, in 1809 and, 25 years after her death, it was joined with the European community. It began a health care ministry at the Baltimore Infirmary, now the University of Maryland Hospital, in 1823.

Thomas Sebastian Byrne, fifth Catholic bishop of the diocese of Nashville, conceived the idea for a hospital operated by the order. Financier Thomas W. Wrenne shrewdly advised him not to make a public announcement

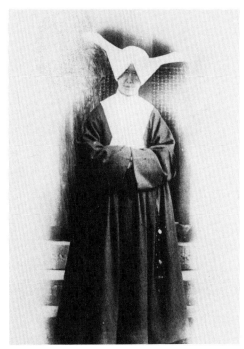

Sister Scholastica Kehoe, a trained pharmacist, she served as president of St. Thomas's board of directors from 1904 to 1927

lest it drive up the costs of potential sites. At the Bishop's request, Wrenne quietly looked at such locations, and recommended the home place of Judge Jacob McGavock Dickinson, at the time assistant attorney general of the United States. It comprised eight acres lying between what is now Hayes and Church streets, and bounded on the north and south by present-day 20th and 21st Avenues, South. "The property is the most beautiful and desirable in Nashville," Bishop Byrne declared. It is "in the most aristocratic portion of the city," a visitor observed.

In December 1897 the bishop wrote to the mother superior of the Daughters of Charity, in Emmitsburg, querying whether they would be interested in help to establish a hospital. "

It is not clear whether the banker and the bishop disclosed their interest to Judge Dickinson in advance. He readily accepted a payment of $50,000, remitted by the "Corporation of St. Joseph's, Emmitsburg," remarking only after that they had got the property at "a very cheap price."

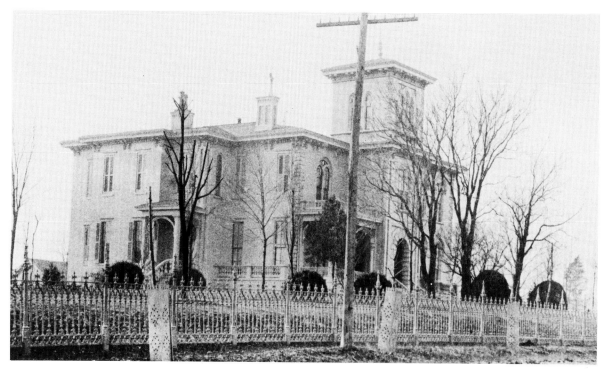

Residence of Jacob McGavock Dickinson

He vacated his former home on March 1, 1898, and that same day sisters from the Daughters of Charity arrived to begin converting it to temporary quarters for the hospital, which would be named for Bishop Byrnes' patron saint, the apostle Thomas. It opened on Easter Monday, April 11.

A year later, these quarters were strained to capacity—33 patients—and the sisters embarked on a campaign to build an entire new hospital. They won endorsements from physicians of the town, and more importantly active help in soliciting funds. Dr. William L. Dudley, dean of the medical department of Vanderbilt, served as chairman of the fundraising committee. His letterhead asking for contributions included the name of Thomas Wrenne and other leaders from the social and financial elite of Nashville.

Even in these prosperous years, the cost of $100,000 to build a central section was slow to come by. The Dickinson home served as St. Thomas hospital for four years. On

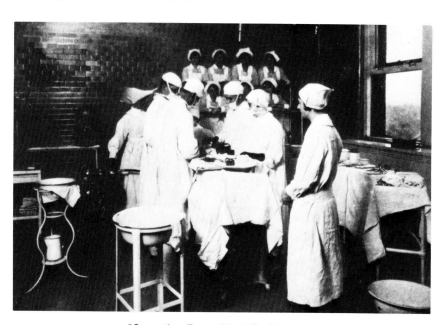

"Operating Room No. 7," mid-1920s

January 29, 1902, the Governor of Tennessee, the Mayor of Nashville, the Chancellor of Vanderbilt University, and other such personages gathered to speechify at the grand opening of the new facility. Visitors looked into the rooms and ward, where 150 patients could be received, and examined the new equipment ready for use.

A new surgical building, between the hospital and the

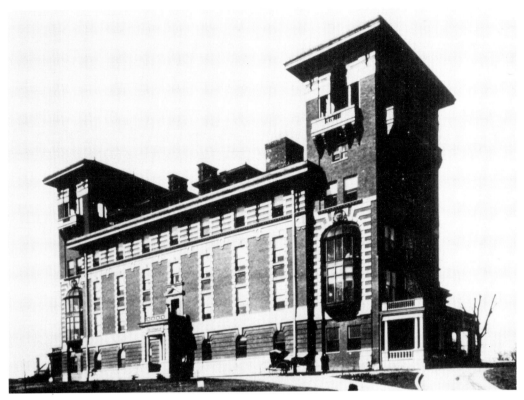

The new St. Thomas Hospital, 1902

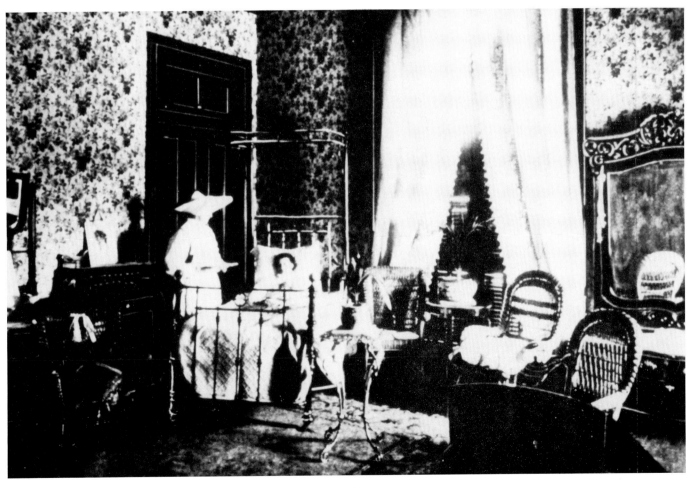

Bruton Room

Dickinson mansion, had two operating rooms, sterilizing room, instrument room, and amenities. Surgery's central place in the new hospitals of Nashville and the world was symbolized by sumptuous decor, including wainscotted Italian marble, six feet high. Despite debts still owed for the Dickinson property, the sisters had not felt the need to economize here. In the center was an ampitheatre where five hundred students could watch Nashville surgeons demonstrate their art.

St. Thomas threw down a challenge to—and offered an alternative for— the infirmary movement of doctors. The new facility provided a place where the therapeutic advances of medicine were being introduced, both in surgery, and against the contagious diseases like typhoid, tuberculosis and diphtheria. The proprietors of such clinics now had the option of a popularly-received hospital setting. In 1905 Dr. Haggard closed his private clinic and transferred his patients to the new hospital. Historians of the institution claimed it was the first time a local doctor

turned to a hospital for the care of patients who could not return home soon after surgery. Acute treatment and convalescence here converged.

Following Dr. Haggard's affiliation, St. Thomas soon recruited to its staff other prominent doctors like Lucius Burch, A. W. Harris, Duncan Eve, Sr., Harrison Shoulders, and others. The last, a future president of the American Medical Association, may have been the first medical student serving an internship at the hospital.

St. Thomas began its renowned nursing school in 1902, housed in the Dickinson mansion. The three-year course comprised "lecture, study, and daily practice in the sickroom," according to announcments from the time. On January 20, 1905, the first class graduated.

New additions went up in the years of the World War, including a building to house the nursing school and a wing perpendicular to the original building on the west side. It fronted today's 21st Avenue North, at the corner of Hayes Street.

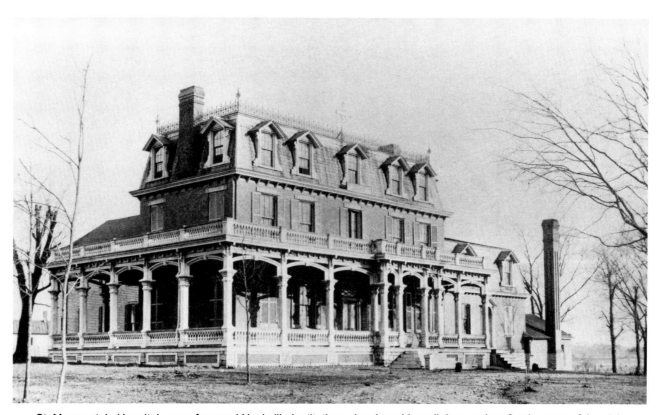

St. Margarete's Hospital, one of several Nashville institutions developed by religious orders for the care of the sick

PROTESTANT AND BAPTIST HOSPITALS

On March 22, 1919 the doors officially opened at Protestant Hospital, situated on the old homestead of Samuel Murphy on Church Street near 20th Avenue, South. Two days earlier, an expectant mother, Gladys Kilby, became the first patient. A few hours later, Margaret Anita Kilby was born.

This institution was planned by the Ministers' Alliance of Nashville. Among the principals involved in the effort were Leslie Cheek (son of coffee magnate Joel Cheek), Dr. Ryland Knight, George Stowe, Dr. E. M. Sanders, and Dr. Rufus E. Fort.

Published reports declared that the Protestant churches of the city would have an equal voice in the management and no physician would ever be named to the board of governors. In addition to paying patients, the hospital planned to care for a number of charity cases, sent by the churches.

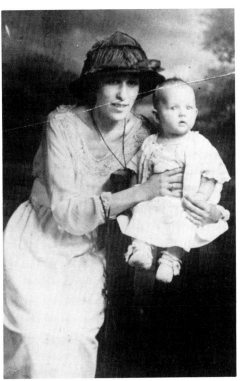
Baptist Hospital's first two patients, Gladys Kilby and her daughter Margaret Anita Kilby Lewis, born on March 20, 1919.

Nearly a quarter of a million dollars was spent on the building and equipment, and space was available for about 100 patients. In 1924 these proprietors added another wing, including patient rooms, a unit for newborns, and surgical theater. Bed capacity stood at 210.

From that original five-acre site eventually rose the great campus of Baptist Hospital. The Southern Baptist Convention had opened a hospital in 1930, on the northwest corner of present-day Eighth Avenue North at Union Street. But Tennessee, the South, and the nation were sinking into the Great Depression. Hospitals, like financial institutions, joined forces to save themselves. Baptist and the Protestant Hospital merged, consolidating with them Dozier Hospital which had served patients in north Nashville. The move availed the new institution nothing. Three years later, in the depths of the crisis, the hospital went into receivership. Revival of the institution would await a more prosperous postwar world.

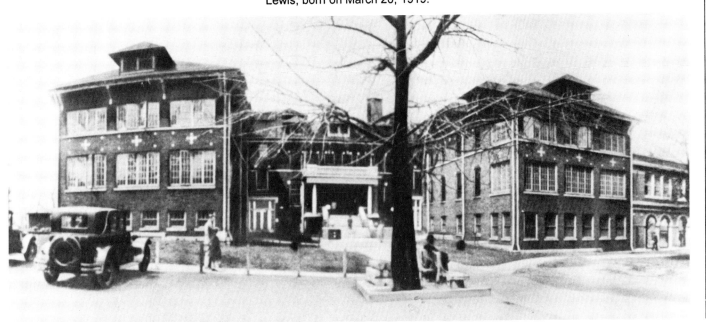
The Protestant Hospital, the original building of Baptist Hospital, about 1930.

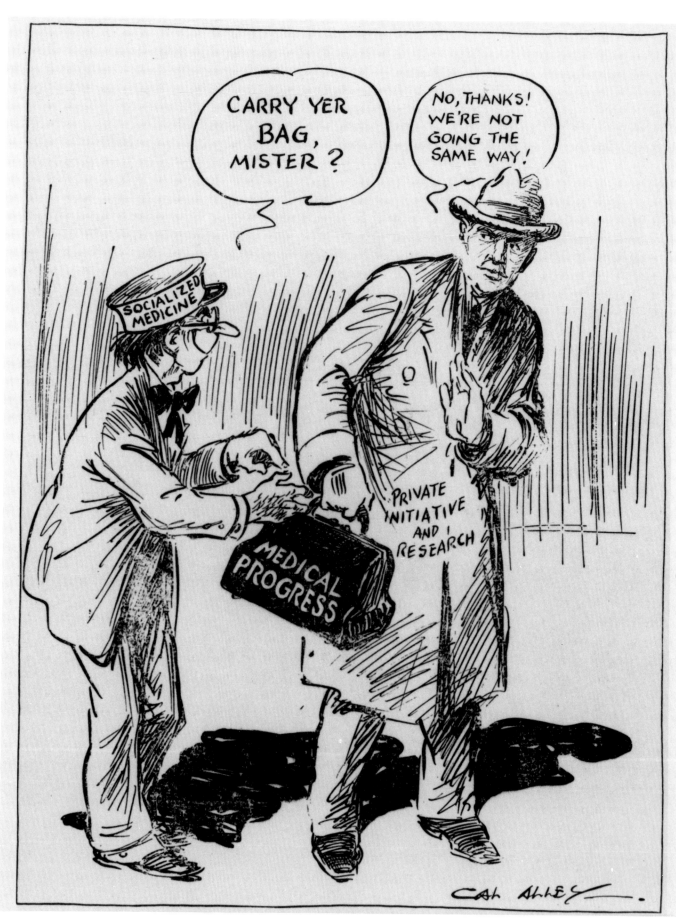

Physicians wary of an overweening government role in medicine had a friend in the publisher's office at the *Nashville Banner*. This cartoon by Cal Alley appeared in that newspaper on March 6, 1944.

Chapter Seven

THE STRUGGLE FOR AUTONOMY

Some 350 physicians were practicing in the city when the nation went to war in April, 1917. More than 100 of them entered the army or navy medical corps. Others received commissions but were unable to go; some of the Nashville doctors' applications were rejected by the War Department on the grounds that they were needed at home. The physicians who remained behind were left to cope with the local effects of the influenza pandemic that spread around the world in 1918 and 1919.

Ironically, the plague struck a city that new standards of sanitation, public health, and pure food and drug laws had helped free from contagious illness. The old nemesis of childhood, diphtheria, plunged after physicians had the antitoxin. Smallpox yielded to a vaccine. Typhoid also gave way before immunization, as well as better understanding of how it was transmitted.

But the mobilization for war had revealed a citizenry beset by significant health problems and deficiencies. One recruit in three was found to be physically unfit for service. Six generic problems led sixty-five percent of all rejections:

- diseases of heart and blood vessels (13.1%)
- deformities and diseases of bones and joints (12.3%)
- errors of vision and diseases of the eye (10.6%)
- mental and nervous disorders and deficiencies (10.3%)
- tuberculosis (9.6%), and
- developmental defects (8.4%)

Nashville physician Paul DeWitt asked some searching questions about these statistics. "Why is the youth of the land so afflicted by heart lesions? Is the high percentage of bone and joint deformities unavoidable, or is it due partly to lack of careful and skillful handling of fractures and diseases by physicians and surgeons?" As for mental and nervous disorders, he observed, "Illiteracy and ignorance stalk through this land of enlightenment and education, and neurasthenics seem to be becoming more numerous." And he added, "The great white plague [tuberculosis] continues its ravages uncontrolled. . . ." Some of Dr. DeWitt's colleagues lamented high the incidence of venereal disease. Dr. A. Frank Richards, president of the state medical association, called prophylactic stations in large cities "one of the greatest and most crying needs of civilization" and a work that organized medicine should undertake.

LIFELONG MEDICAL LEARNING

Most leaders of organized medicine, in Nashville and throughout the nation, acknowledged although older members of the profession had earned a diploma in a rigorous medical curriculum, the discovery of new knowledge was outpacing that preparation. Dr. William Osler in an address before the New Haven Medical Association in 1903 declared:

> "We doctors do not take stock often enough,
> and are very apt to carry on our shelves stale,
> out-of-date goods."

He went on to note that participation in a medical society helped a physician to "furnish his mental shop with the latest wares. Rightly used, it may be a touchstone to which he can bring his experiences to the test and save him from falling into a few sequences."

To acknowledge that fact did not connote disrespect for the previous generation of physicians. It merely recognized that one with the medical education of the 1890s would think differently than the graduate of the 1920s. As the *Journal of the Tennessee State Medical Association* observed in 1919, "We still have an unduly large number of pulse and tongue diagnosticators and an unduly large number of symptom treaters."

The Nashville Academy of Medicine attempted to provide Oslerian touchstones, inviting a paper at each of its meetings, followed by discussion. On the statewide level, the Tennessee State Medical Association offered scientific sessions at its annual meetings. Edited by a succession of Nashville physicians, its *Journal* offered articles, case reports, and scientific abstracts in specialty subjects. The same editorial cited above continued, ". .

.The men in the profession who are using scientific methods in diagnosis and who have gotten away from blind prescribing for presenting symptoms are far more numerous than they were ten, or even five, years ago."

Postgraduate education moved to the top of the agenda of medical societies during the 1920s and 1930s. The Nashville Academy of Medicine mounted one of the earliest efforts to keep local doctors current by establishing a fund to bring outstanding speakers from out of town to give lectures and demonstrations. In the spring of 1921 the Tennessee Section of the American College of Surgeons gave its first clinical session in Nashville, providing clinics in four hospitals over two days.

By the 1930s the two medical schools had also begun paying attention to the need of lifelong learning among alumni. Within just a few years after the school's opening, the Vanderbilt University Medical Society offered rich and popular programs. In 1936 Meharry began a postgraduate seminar in its School of Nursing and a formal postgraduate course in medicine that expanded in the postwar years into full-fledged training for advanced academic degrees.

With help from the Commonwealth Fund, the state medical association began, in 1937, offering courses in 10 teaching circuits across the state. Each of these circuits had five centers, and the same lecture was given every week in each center, after being publicized by mail and through county medical societies.

Obstetrics was chosen as the subject most needed, since its problems presented themselves to every physician in general practice. An observer of these early days noted that as a result doctors were being invited to speak to women's clubs, parent-teachers associations, and especially girls of high-school age on the causes and methods of prevention of maternal deaths. "Although this is only the first step," wrote Dr. Frank Whitacre, "prenatal care will come into its own and regular visits to the doctor during pregnancy will result. In this regard Tennessee may well consider herself a pioneer."

In time courses were offered in pediatrics, internal

medicine, surgical diagnosis, and gynecology. Lectures were followed or preceded by clinical demonstrations and doctors were encouraged to request consultations on their private cases. The state society revised the project in 1955, and began offering symposia, presented on a specific topic by several physician-instructors. The symposia were then scheduled three times a year in each of ten districts.

Leadership of the postgraduate movement was strongly urban, and names of prominent Nashville physicians are found on the state medical association's organizing committees. However, attendance at the programs was poor in the cities, and by the early 1960s, presenting physicians found themselves speaking to sparse audiences. For a few years, organized medicine in Tennessee withdrew from the endeavor, but Vanderbilt, the University of Tennessee, and Meharry all began courses aimed mainly at general practitioners.

Just as the Tennessee society found its program faltering, the AMA nationally took up the cause of lifelong learning for doctors, now called "continuing education." By the end of the 1960s, the AMA began recognizing physicians who assumed responsibility for their own programs of study, and the state association offered to act as a liaison between community hospitals and medical societies to encourage doctors to attend cliniopathological conferences and go on rounds. The AMA would first certify those institutions found capable of offering substantive programs of continuing education (versus "sitting and dozing"). In 1974, the state association won approval from the AMA's Committee on Medical Education to approve these certifications on its own.

The development of Tennessee's modern system of continuing medical education, growing up and out from

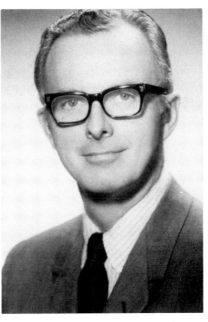

Dr. Tom E. Nesbitt, who served as president of the American Medical Association in 1978

the circuit-riding and symposia days, included leadership from Nashville doctors Rudolph H. Kampmeier, Robert Roy, John B. Thomison, Fred D. Ownby, Tom E. Nesbitt, Frank A. Perry, Paul E. Slaton, and C. K. Meador.

COSTS AND DISTRIBUTION

The partnership with science was paying huge dividends in the old quest for "what worked." There were the liver extracts, and insulin that controlled diabetes in the 1920s. Infectious diseases, one of humanities' great banes, were tamed by the sulfonamides, introduced in the 1930s. Veteran Nashville plastic surgeon Greer Ricketson recalled how parents had once resisted repair of such woes as cleft palate and congenital deformities, arguing that what God had made should not be disturbed. Yet surgical repair, although done at high risk, was being successfully reported in the *Journal* of the Tennessee Medical Association by 1930, just one of the rapid advances in that specialty.

Thus grew the public's belief that health problems once faced with stoic resignation could now be treated, relieved, cured. The press wrote of "miracle drugs" and "magic bullets," but this popular explosion of confidence in medicine had several consequences.

First, it coincided with the reforms in medical education now taking effect after a generation of concerted work by organized medicine capturing and applying state power. The numbers of doctors in Tennessee plummeted, as requirements to study medicine, graduate, and win a license became stiffer. These fewer doctors had more respect and higher incomes, but also higher expectations placed on them.

The public now wanted more of medicine's promises; the doctors naturally enjoyed their new prestige and wanted to protect such prerogatives as they had won. But this market situation—more patients seeking fewer physicians—tended to inflate the cost of seeing a doctor. At the same time, in Tennessee, the press took note of the uneven distribution of physicians. From time to time lawmakers and editorial writers in Tennessee and elsewhere expressed concern about an alleged insufficiency of doctors in rural areas. Indeed physicians were drawn to cities, where new hospitals gave them opportunities for service and professional advancement.

The higher bills to patients and fewer physicians in some locales set off widespread worry. In response, a privately funded commission formed in 1926 to study the nation's health care system. The Committee on the Costs of Medical Care, as it was called, became one of the most important bodies in the making of modern health policy in the United States. Members included economists, physicians, and public health specialists, many of whom supported mandatory health insurance.

For the next five years, staff compiled a vast library of research about medical care. It found, generally, that nearly half of well-to-do families surveyed received medical care during the course of a year, while over 40 percent of lowest-income families did not. The burden of the system also lay on people who paid the most. The 3.5 percent of families with the highest medical bills paid one third of the cost of all medical care in the country.

Two essential assumptions lay at the heart of all those research reports. First, medical care was the business of doctors. It noted illnesses that might have had their origins in poor nutrition, or substandard housing, or a dangerous work place. Yet medical care "can be defined only in terms of the physical conditions of the people and the capacities of the science and art of medicine to deal with them."

The committee also decided that practically everybody, even the affluent, needed more medical services. Accordingly, the nation ought to spend more of its national resources on medical care. The committee's final report endorsed group practice and group payment for medical care, but opposed compulsory health insurance.

As for low-income people, local governments should contribute a share of the costs of group payment plans, "assisted where necessary by state and federal governments."

A minority report written by eight private practitioners on the committee urged that government get out of medicine entirely—except for the care of the indigent, who should become its responsibility. This strident document rejected not only mandatory health insurance, but voluntary private insurance as well, since these were "a longer or shorter bridge to a compulsory system." Organized medicine endorsed this minority report, and won considerable press coverage about the threat of "socialized medicine." In consequence, the incoming administration of Franklin D. Roosevelt shied away from even modest proposals for changing how people might pay for their medical bills.

Nashville physician Olin West served as the American Medical Association's representative to the Committee on the Costs of Medical Care. In 1933 he came home and gave a first-hand report on the panel's work. He castigated the panel as coming from big cities ("that great artificiality and monstrosity") and for a staff that comprised doctors of philosophy rather than doctors of medicine. Although this staff knew nothing about what was involved in serving people, they had criticized the profession as "static and unprogressive."

"STATE MEDICINE"

There followed a great struggle, in Nashville, in Tennessee, and throughout the nation, over government's role in medicine. Doctors had invited state power into their realm, as seen in the campaign for licensure standards guaranteed by law. Before that, sanitation regulation backed by legal sanction had first given the profession an entree into the public realm.

Early in the twentieth century, Tennessee doctors still saw a need for state assistance to medicine for public health and charitable care-giving. Dr. A. Frank Richards,

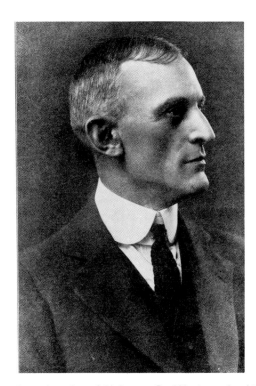

Dr. Olin West. A native of Alabama, Dr. West received the M.D. degree from Vanderbilt University in 1899. He began his career as smallpox inspector for the Nashville City Board of Health and was later the executive officer for the Tennessee State Board of Health. In 1922 he joined the staff of the American Medical Association and was elected its president in 1948.

president of the state medical association, called for establishing city and county health departments to enforce sanitary laws and regulations. for better reporting by doctors of births, and other powers to the state for public health. Dr. L. L. Shadden, another state association president, called for provision of facilities for indigent tuberculosis patients, a state home for "mental defectives," and a hospital fund for the benefit of children born with deformities.

On the national scene, Franklin D. Roosevelt's "New Deal" undertook a vast expansion of the federal presence in the field of public health. Congress passed the Maternal and Child Health Act and made increasing amounts of money available to state and local health agencies. The appropriations for the United States Public Health Service also swelled year after year, with sizable allocations to state health departments for program expansion, training of personnel, and research. The 1937 Housing Act,

supported by the American Public Health Association, provided for slum clearance ("urban renewal" as the euphemism had it) in metropolitan areas. The following spring, lawmakers enacted the Venereal Disease Act, which promoted prevention and treatment of maladies once unmentionable in polite company. In a single year alone, 1938-39, the number of clinics for diagnosis and treatment of venereal diseases increased by more than thirty per cent around the nation. Industrial hygiene received new public attention when a division devoted to it was set up at the National Institutes of Health in 1935.

When local, state, and federal government actually attempted to shoulder some tasks proposed by Drs. Richards and Shadden, other physicians rebelled. To give them their intellectual honesty, they sought to make a division of labor between state agencies engaged in promoting good health practices among the general population and doctors giving direct patient care. Dr. Harrison Shoulders, who became one of Nashville's presidents of the American Medical Association (1946-47), took up the cause of professional autonomy when, in the Thirties, he led opposition to government-funded hospitals for veterans of the first World War. As editor of the journal of the state medical association he for many years printed on its masthead:

THE ISSUE
SHALL PATIENTS AND DOCTORS RETAIN
THEIR FREEDOM OF JUDGMENT
IN THE MATTER OF MEDICAL CARE,
OR SHALL THIS FREEDOM BE SURRENDERED
TO SOME GOVERNMENTAL AGENCY?

Dr. Shoulders saw public health departments as state subsidy of parental neglect; mothers and fathers should take their child to a private practitioner for inoculations and other needs. For like-minded physicians, the struggle came to a head when the profession lost control over the Tennessee Department of Public Health. Before 1923 it had been under the State Board of Public Health, comprising three doctors and the Commissioner of Agriculture,

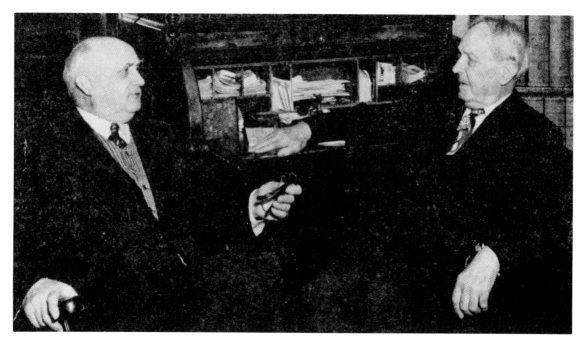

Drs. Harrison Shoulders, left, and William H. Witt

all appointed by the governor. That year Governor Austin Peay won passage in the General Assembly of a bill restructuring cabinet departments and state agencies. It abolished the Board of Health and placed the Department of Health under a Commissioner who had complete authority to establish all its policies and regulations.

During the next ten years or so, the organized medical profession and the department gradually became estranged. The state medical association sought legislation to reestablish the Board of Health and to include six physicians and one dentist. The governor would still appoint, but only from nominees submitted by the state medical and dental associations. The effort failed in the General Assembly.

The profession conceded that it hoped that the state would not furnish "unrestricted [medical] service to any who might apply." In the legislature sitting in the winter of 1935, physicians came back. Organized under Dr. John M. Lee of Nashville, they won backing of a departmental reorganization bill from every county medical society except one, and secured pledges of support from 30 of 33 elected members of the Senate and 82 of 98 elected members of the House of Representatives.

It achieved a further legislative triumph that same session by successfully lobbying for a measure that provided that members of the State Board of Medical Examiners would be appointed by the governor from nominees certified by the society, rather than by purely gubernatorial choice.

It was an achievement comparable to that of 1889, when public health doctors, arguing their case for being able to do real good to people, took their authority as conclusive over all of medicine's realm and won a licensure law, a monopoly, in effect. Here the profession kept control over state medicine by insisting that doctors—and not representatives from lay groups or successful politicians—should pass on treating people, either for illness or prevention. Dr. W. C. Williams, state commissioner of public health, worked a synthesis. He called for the public health worker and "we of the organized medical profession" to resist the changes in the practices of medicine . . . or "be engulfed in a reform wave of social and economic hysteria." The public health regulations enforced by his department would in the future be promulgated by the State Board of Health. His department would stress prevention of the diseases ravaging Tennessee people: tuberculosis, diphtheria, syphilis, typhoid fever, malaria. In all this—and in promising central services like diagnostic laboratories, analysis of local water supplies, and establishment of a full-time health service in every county—he pledged cooperation and consultation with county medical societies.

Dr. Lee concluded that the interests of the state and private practitioners were now aligned, and gave his blessing. By the mid-1950s, the department was greatly expanding its budget and in the direction of causes and concerns of physicians of the 1930s and 1940s: money to cover the costs of hospitalization for indigent Tennesseans; enlarging the battle against tuberculosis; and a program designed to reduce the crippling effects caused by rheumatic fever and congenital heart disease.

Tennessee doctors also responded to the criticism that medicine had become too expensive for poor people. In the mid-1930s, reporters and editorial writers in Tennessee and elsewhere raised questions about the equity and justice of some people being able to afford health care and others not. Medical societies set up delivery of care, especially hospital care, under plans that enabled the patient to settle his bill in installments. In 1943, Dr. John Owsley Manier of Nashville took chairmanship of a state medical association committee on prepayment plans for hospital and medical services. The panel recommended the Blue Cross Plan for Prepayment Hospitalization and urged the Tennessee State Hospital Association to adopt it.

Dr. Manier's committee sounded the tocsin: unless the medical profession and the hospitals convinced the public that they "offered the best possible service in the world regardless of income," the federal government would take

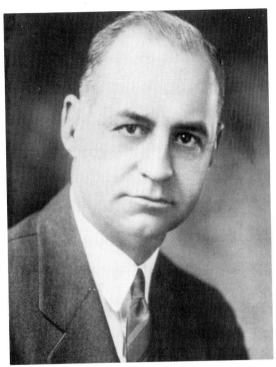
Dr. John Owsley Manier

control over the practice of medicine.

Lingering concern over rising cost of care may have contributed to the temporary weakening of organized medicine's great triumph in Tennessee, the 1889 law that regulated medical practice in the state, and the subsequent amendments that made it more stringent. With some 600 physicians away in wartime service, the General Assembly sitting in 1943 admitted naturopaths to the practice of medicine in Tennessee (joining physicians and surgeons, osteopaths, and chiropractors). During the next eighteen months, some one thousand such practitioners received a license. In the spring of 1945, organized medicine regained the political initiative and persuaded legislators to pass the Basic Sciences Law requiring all persons seeking to practice any healing art to stand examination in anatomy, chemistry, physiology, bacteriology, and pathology. Two years later, it won repeal of the naturopathy act altogether.

THE TRIUMPH OF PUBLIC SERVICE

Even as the leadership of organized medicine felt threatened by "state medicine," medical societies urged members to assume responsibility for immunizing children against diphtheria, smallpox, and typhoid. Public service became the watchword of the Nashville Academy of Medicine and the state medical association in the late 1940s and early 1950s, as doctors bent on protecting their hard-won privileges decided public relations campaigns might help. In the postwar years, the Nashville Academy of Medicine placed on its agenda a range of community concerns, reminiscent of the old-time when sanitarians first made valid claims for what medicine could do.

Nashville physician Leonard Wright ("Win") Edwards led the state medical association's committee on public service, established in 1950, coming to the post after a long struggle against "state medicine." As chairman of the legislative committee (i.e., chief lobbyist) he was credited as a major force in the passage of the Basic Science law. In 1939 he won passage in the General Assembly an act creating the medical care division of the state Department of Public Health, which provided that federal funds for medical care would come through and be regulated by this agency.

In 1953 the Tennessee General Assembly created a program to provide for hospital care for low-income people. It was driven in part by the inability of urban general hospitals to absorb poor people from surrounding counties, brought there for care because their local hospital made no provision for paying the bills. This indigent hospitalization program was created by the public service committee of the state medical association, which panel was led by Nashville doctors. Under the statute, a state appropriation was allocated to each county. In the first year of operation more than two-thirds of the state's 95 counties had adopted the plan. Crafted by physicians, it was also administered by them: doctors reviewed the cases of persons seeking hospitalization as indigents, decided the need, and chose the hospital. Administrators in the state public health department only made sure that fiscal regulations were followed and paperwork done properly.

The state society's public service committee became its most influential one by the early 1950s. Its executive subcommittee comprised three Nashville doctors, Dr. Edwards, Dr. Charles C. Trabue, IV, and Dr. John Owsley Manier. The association established friendly relations with reporters and editors of national magazines, produced television programs and documentary films, sponsored an annual medical education week, and undertook numerous other endeavors. For a time these were directed by young Jesse Hill Ford, Jr., later famous as the author of *The Liberation of Lord Byron Jones* and other novels.

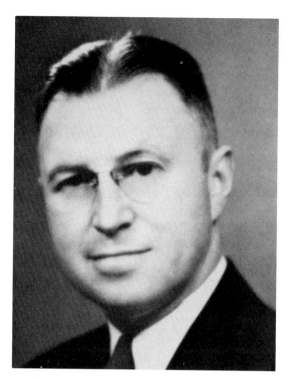

Dr. Leonard W. Edwards, aggressive leader of the Tennessee State Medical Association's public service campaign.

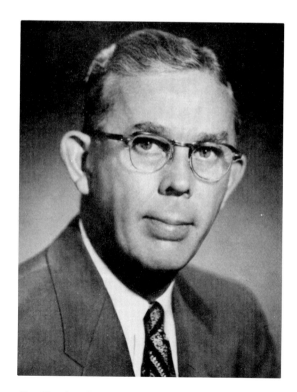

Dr. Charles C. Trabue, IV. Dr. Trabue was great-grandson of Charles C. Trabue who served as mayor of Nashville in 1839

THE YOUNGEST PATIENTS

In 1921 Congress passed the Shepherd-Towner Act, which authorized matching funds to the every state for health centers serving pregnant women and children. Staffing the centers, public health nurses and women physicians offered advice to expectant mothers about how to avoid common illnesses associated with carrying a baby and caring for it in early life. As private physicians took up an interest in these tasks, the AMA could argue the law was unneeded, and Congress repealed it in 1927.

The interest in maternal and child welfare was genuine and far-reaching on the part of Nashville and Tennessee doctors. County societies made these subjects a theme of their program each May (in connection with Mothers Day). By the late 1930s doctors were studying the incidence of infant mortality in the state and the causes, with prematurity found as a big factor. Dr. J. Owsley Manier noted in 1935 that little sustained improvement had been had in morbidity and mortality from diphtheria over ten years, despite press acclaim to programs of inoculation by local health departments especially among young school-children. Had assumptions by the state of providing this and prophylactics against smallpox and typhoid been necessary? He grudgingly conceded that it had. Despite advice from doctors, the public by and large had been slow to appreciate the need for the therapeutic advances of medicine. A child could have received protection at an earlier age—if parents had seen their doctor and asked. In his outgoing address as president of the state medical association, Dr. Manier pledged that it would send speakers to every county medical society in the state to demonstrate methods of immunization, and it called upon the State Board of Health to assist with the program. Later on, he added, the society would carry down to the local groups "advanced knowledge on such matters as infant welfare, prenatal maternal care, the cancer problem, tuberculosis, the venereal problem, periodic health examinations," and

other matters. He continued, "If the medical profession wishes to control such problems, we must handle them ourselves, or else ill-informed lay organizations will take them in hand . . . ."

In a comprehensive survey of Tennessee public schools in 1946, the State Department of Education found that "health" was the most desirable objective that Tennesseeans thought the schools could help pupils achieve. The agency considered that this involved physical education, health instruction, health services, school lunches, and safety. It called on the medical societies in each county to lend advice and counsel to superintendents, who were responsible for all school health programs.

Tennessee's children with disabilities began receiving special attention in 1919, when Dr. Willis Campbell, a Memphis orthopaedic surgeon persuaded a local charity to establish the Crippled Children's Hospital School there. A fellow specialist in Nashville, Dr. Adam Nichol, interested the Junior League in the subject and in the fall of 1923 the Junior League Home for Crippled Children opened in the city.

Eleemosynary organizations, especially the Tennessee Society for Crippled Children and the Rotary Club, took up the banner, and in 1929 the State of Tennessee entered the realm in 1929 with an appropriation for such work. In 1937 the Crippled Children's Service was established in the Tennessee Department of Public Health, and it grew in responsibility, backed by orthopaedists, plastic surgeons, and other physicians.

Two years later, the world went to war again, and Nashville's children were put at risk. The 1943 annual report of the Department of Health show a sharp increase in infant deaths that year. Epidemiologists attributed this rise to children being left at home unattended, their fathers gone to war, their mothers working night and day in the city's roaring factories to make production and meet contract deadlines.

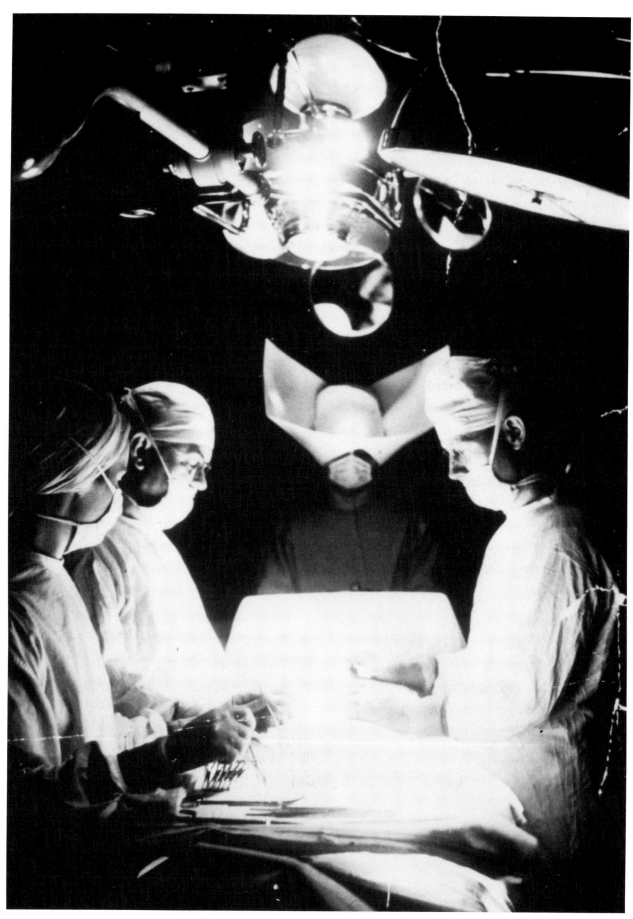

Surgery at St. Thomas Hospital during a simulated city-wide blackout in 1942.
Left is Dr. James D. Lester. His colleague is Dr. Sidney Ballard.

Chapter Eight

WAR AND POSTWAR CHANGE

ollowing the Japanese attack on Pearl Harbor, a kind of hysteria spread over the nation, and the city. Although
they lived deep inland, many Nashvillians expected air raids and the injuries they were sure to inflict. The local
Civilian Defense Council assumed responsibility for preparing Nashville to cope with bombing and readied for
blackouts, organized emergency crews, and appointed decontamination teams. The CDC also trained citizens in
emergency medicine. People were taught how to defuse bombs and give basic first aid for trauma. A nurse's aide course
at Hubbard Hospital trained black Nashvillians, and the Red Cross started what it claimed was the "first Negro unit"
in the nation, an intensive 80-hour course in coping with the war when it came home.

Nashville doctors answered the call to make certain that would not happen. By November 1942, 160 of Davidson
County's 220 physicians were gone, to take up a rifle, command a unit, or to manage a part of the apparatus of
mobilization. Vanderbilt's Hugh Morgan accepted a major assignment in the office of the U. S. Surgeon General. John

Youmans succeeded him as acting chairman of the
Department of Medicine but left in the winter of
1944 to direct the Surgeon General's nutrition
corps.

Teaching, training, and research at the city's two
medical schools took a severe buffeting. Half of the
senior faculty in medicine at Vanderbilt had left for
military duty by the fall of 1943. Some of them
joined with the dean, Dr. Morgan, to form the 300th
General Hospital Unit, which saw service in North
Africa and Italy.

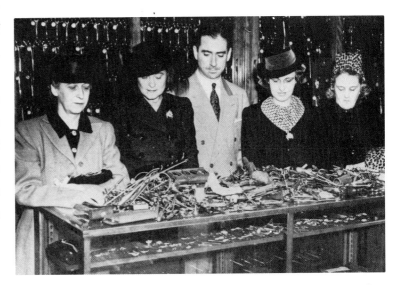

Nashville physicians contributed more than 700 surgical instruments for shipment to England so colleagues there
could treat victims of Nazi air raids. Assisting with this "Bundles for Britain" drive in 1940 were, left to right, Mrs.
Pringle Rhett, Mrs. Robert Webster, Mr. Dan Maddox, Mrs. John Fenner Cummins, and Mrs. Newman Cheek.

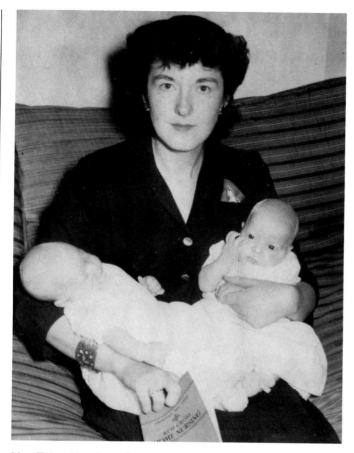

Mrs. Taber Hamilton, Jr. keeps a home nursing manual close at hand as a guide in the care of her two-month-old twin daughters, Sydney Graves (left) and Virginia Walker Hamilton. Mrs. Hamilton was one of many Nashville mothers enrolled in home nursing instruction courses during the wartime nurse and physician shortage.

"The war ravaged medical education at Vanderbilt," recalled Dr. Samuel Riven years later. Dr. Rudolph Kampmeier, senior full-time person in the department of medicine, faced a continuous parade of students, interns and residents, a shortage of key personnel, and constant demands for maintenance on the physical plant, for which he had no money. He formed himself and five part-timers into three teams, rotating their assignments every trimester. One would be assigned to the wards and the other two to the outpatient department. Classes, ward rounds, and clinics passed in a dizzying round. "It was hard and bleak," said Dr. Riven, "and before it was over strained friendships, and nerves, and family life." Yet Dr. Kampmeier could modestly observe, in his memoirs, that "the Department of Medicine fulfilled its responsibilities reasonably well."

Meharry's fighting men also went off to the fronts. The school had to do more and more with less and less, as it went to an accelerated program in which new first year classes were admitted every nine months. Operations were year-round, so that the faculty could cover four years' work in three—but the number of these teachers declined each month. Those that remained were mainly part-time, earning their livelihood in private practice.

As in 1862-65, venereal disease followed the armies to Nashville. Millions of soldiers swarmed through on weekends from the nearby bases. By late 1942, as many as 80,000 of them could be found in town on any given weekend. Civic organizations and private volunteers promoted their wholesome accommodations and hospitality—but honky-tonks and prostitutes by the hundreds offered a beer and a friendly pair of arms. Seen in one way, it was another economic boon of the war, as long-time hookers and eager young girls, some of high school age, took advantage of lonely Army men, far from home, with cash to spend. By day the women who took men's place on the production line at Vultee turned out the planes to beat Hitler. By night, others offered a few hours' consolation to boys on their way to the Pacific islands. As a

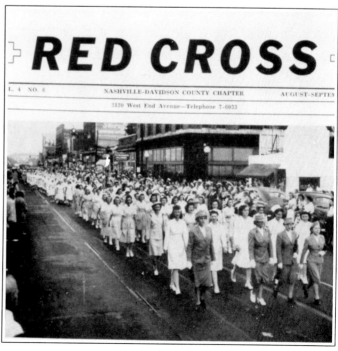

The Red Cross Section of the V-J Day Parade, Eighth and Broadway, 1945.

result syphilis and gonorrhea spread like wildfire. Infection rates were so high by 1942 that Washington invoked a measure that made vice activity near military bases a federal offense, called for severe sentences for prostitutes, and enlisted the Federal Bureau of Investigation in antiprostitution efforts.

The City Health Department, which had grown through the strained Depression years, now mushroomed. In 1942 it operated one venereal disease control clinic; the next year, there were six. Syphilis cases grew from 1,200 to 3,500 in that period. The city health budget for venereal disease control tripled during the war years. It was to little avail. The problem grew increasingly worse. Police shut down saloons where prostitutes and their johns were said to meet. Dr. Murray Brown, director of the Nashville venereal disease control program, presented a talk before the Academy of Medicine in the fall of 1943 reporting on the intensive-case finding activities of state and local health departments. He noted two census tracts of the inner city with spectacularly high rates of infection. Investigation revealed that the Army convoys parked there and soldiers given liberty to walk about seeking amusement. He urged that other parking areas be found, where wholesome recreation for soldiers could be found. Nonetheless, high rates of these diseases continued through V-J Day and for years beyond.

An ironic positive outcome was the prestige and sizable budgets enjoyed by the health departments of both city and county government. In the 1940s, the city spent more money on its general hospital: its budget grew by 180 percent. The cause of cleaner streets got an increase of 122 percent, while related programs nearly doubled in their appropriations.

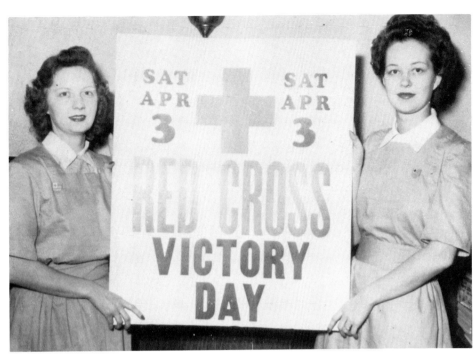

Mrs. Raymond Pirtle, left, and Mrs. Dan Maddox prepare for the Victory Parade on Saturday, April 3, 1943. The two were among 200 women enrolled in home nursing classes that the Red Cross organized throughout the city to meet the wartime shortage of doctors and nurses.

PUBLIC HEALTH AND METROPOLITAN GOVERNMENT

The expansion of Nashville's public health program was part of the expansion of local government generally. The annual budget rose, programs added new agendas and personnel, and city government entered new endeavors like planning and urban renewal. What had been a decided skepticism toward government in the 1930s on the part of citizens generally gave way to favorable reception for an activist city hall. Widespread concern over the city's public health problems freed the city and county departments from narrow and myopic political interests. When they joined together in 1952, it was a harbinger of consolidated city-county government, approved by the voters ten years later.

The establishment of Metropolitan Government in Nashville had roots in a basic problem in public health and sanitation. From the Cumberland River, the city could provide suburbs with abundant supplies of water. Throughout the late 1940s and 1950s, this amenity enabled developers to put up tract housing along curvilinear roads,

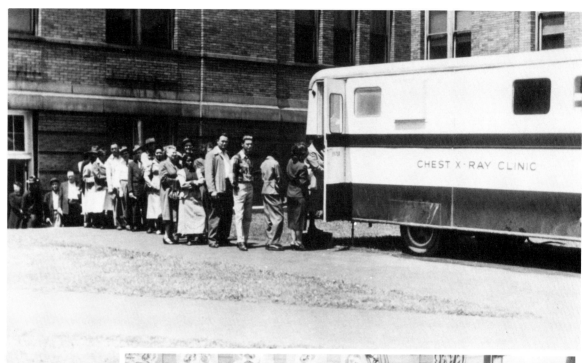

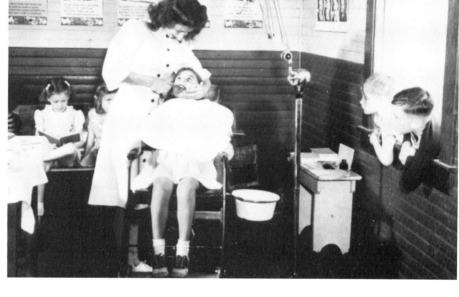

further and further from the old downtown. Another local geological feature countered with a curse: Nashville stood on a base of ancient limestone, which lay from a few inches to a few feet below the soil surface. Sewer lines would come at a high price tag, so homeowners wanting nothing to do with higher taxes happily settled for septic tanks. That meant large lots for drainage, which dispersed density, which meant upward spiraling costs for other utilities, like garbage collection and street lighting, and even fire and police protection.

In 1949 less than half of Nashvillians had sewers; the rest had crude outhouses or septic tanks. These often didn't work very well, and Dr. John J. Lentz, county health officer, regularly warned about the threat of disease from rainwater that percolated from the thin soil to the surface. He called for a single plan of action on the part of both local governments to take care of the problem. The morning newspaper called the matter a "ticking time

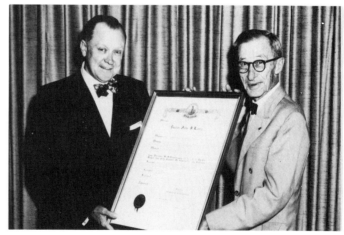

Nashville Mayor Ben West, left, presents an award to Dr. John J. Lentz, director of the Davidson County Health Department for more than 40 years.

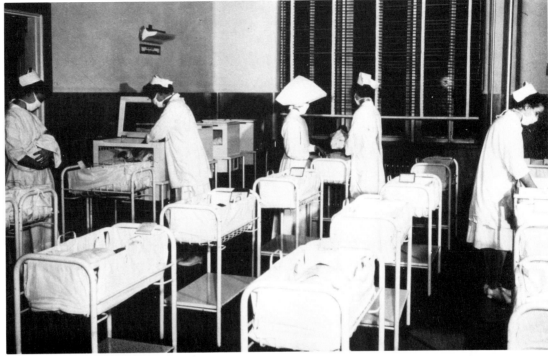

The postwar "baby boom" is already evident in this 1949 photograph of the nursery at St. Thomas Hospital.

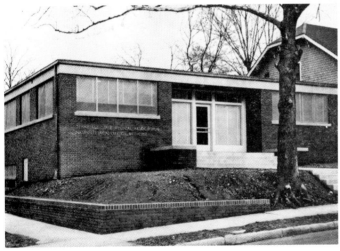

Below: The new home of the Nashville Academy of Medicine and the Tennessee Medical Association, 112 Louise Avenue.

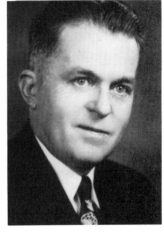

Dr. Daugh W. Smith

been anchored on Church Street, the Public Square, and environs. Dr. Samuel Riven recalled, "Frankly, it was a competitive situation, as far as getting patients."

In the years of postwar prosperity, many physicians were deserting the Doctors Building and Bennie Dillon Building on Church Street and setting up practice around St. Thomas, Baptist, and Vanderbilt. In 1956 The Tennessee Medical Association opened a new headquarters on the corner of Louise Avenue and Hayes Street, in the heart of the area, the building committee comprising Drs. Daugh W. Smith, Charles C. Trabue, IV, and Rudolph H. Kampmeier, all of Nashville. The Nashville Academy of Medicine shared space here until 1974 when it found its own home on nearby 23rd Avenue, North.

By the mid-1990s, the old Murphy tract that the nuns bought a century before had grown to become a sprawling complex of offices for groups and solo practitioners and ancillary health services. It stretched from within a stone's

bomb," but it was to tick for more than a decade, until the Metropolitan Government began addressing the crisis.

The city expanded outward toward every compass point in the 1950s. The first suburban shopping centers sprang up, such as Green Hills, on the old farm lands subdivided from still older plantations. Doctors followed their clients. New medical school graduate, Dr. George B. Hagan looking for a place to establish himself sought out Dr. William Card in Madison, and the pair reached an agreement to practice jointly in a clinic on Gallatin Road.

Hospitals in turn drew doctors to their environs. In the 1930s the commercial and professional life of the city had throw of the old downtown to Centennial Park on the West between West End Avenue to Charlotte Pike. Vanderbilt, too, deliberately drew doctors. Vanderbilt put up the Medical Arts Building on 21st Avenue, South, intending to draw clinical faculty (i.e., its part-time teachers) next door to the school. Medical School dean John Youmans proposed this facility, owned by Vanderbilt and paid for on a self-financing plan. In the years to come, hospitals arranged for physicians' office buildings next door, as they competed for patient admissions. The suburbanization of medical practice became a centrifugal force for the city's second great age of hospital building in the 1970s and beyond.

THE ACADEMY AND MID-CENTURY NASHVILLE

The Academy's ongoing leadership of organized medicine in Tennessee was reflected in its members position as head of key committees of the state medical association. In the mid-1930s, they chaired the panels on scientific work (Dr. Harrison Shoulders), public policy and legislation (Dr. L.W. Edwards), hospitals (Dr. D. R. Pickens), and the liaison committee with the state public health department (Dr. W. C. Dixon). As the state society expanded its agenda, and its board's governing bureaucracy over the next twenty years, the role of Nashville doctors grew. By 1950 eight of 17 committees were under their gavel.

Physicians' engagement with lawmaking naturally meant they met lawyers—in the General Assembly, in public policy committees, and in local leadership circles. In the fall of 1941 the Academy invited the Nashville Bar Association to a fish fry at Hettie Ray's Dinner Club atop Nine Mile Hill. (The locality may be known by that name to anyone age 50 or over; it is the high point on Highway 70 between the present-day Jewish Community

Left: Some of the convalescing soldiers treated at Thayer during the 1940s.

Thayer Veteran's Hospital, on White Bridge Road.

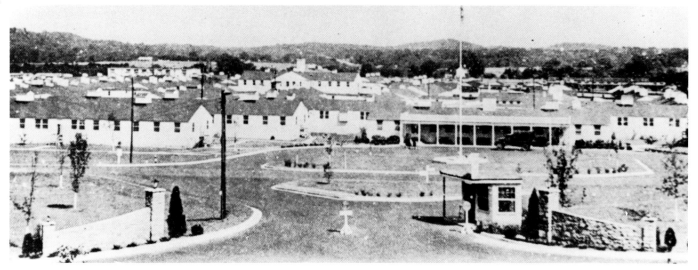

Center and Wessex Towers.) "It is recognized that, as professional men, the two groups have many common interests," observed one reporter. In later years, the cooperation between the two would be embodied in the Academy's standing medico-legal committee.

Although military service thinned the ranks of local doctors, those who stayed home to provide essential service got a realistic demonstration of what their colleagues faced on the battlefield. The Academy convened at Camp [later Fort] Campbell on February 24, 1944, to see a presentation by the camp surgeon, Colonel Herbert E. Taylor, on the successive stages of treatment for soldiers wounded in action. During the war, the academy met twice a month instead of each week. The very state medical enterprises which it distrusted served as hosts occasionally, such as Central State psychiatric hospital and Thayer Veterans Hospital.

Weekly meetings resumed in the fall of 1946, held in the auditorium of the Doctors Building on Church Street. At the annual meeting in January, 1947, Dr. John C. Burch was elected president. In his inaugural address, he put forward a vision that Nashville medicine carried a half-century later.

> All of us are committed to the general principle of developing Nashville as a great medical center. Continuing study is a vital necessity. . .The influence of the Academy in stimulating the professional development of us all is invaluable. Our goal [is] Nashville, the Medical Center of the South.

Some physicians followed the advice of Sir William Osler to never miss a meeting of their medical society. Dr. Rudolph Kampmeier, professor of medicine at Vanderbilt

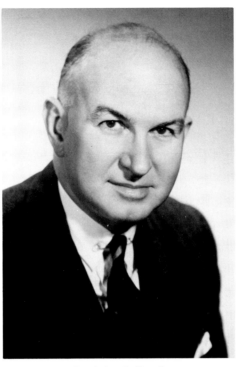

Dr. John C. Burch

and an internist, recalled encountering in the academy's auditorium Dr. Charles C. Trabue, Dr. C. N. Gessler, Irving Hillard, Benjamin Fowler, and Daugh W. Smith. Drs. Trabue, Smith, and Kampmeier would in time serve as presidents of the state medical association. Every student of Tennessee medical history relies on Dr. Kampmeier's history of that organization from 1930 to 1980, a copious compilation of factual information gleaned in part from the TMA *Journal*, which he edited for twenty-one years. He is also remembered as the author of a classical textbook *Physical Examination in Health and Disease* (1950).

In the summer of 1950 the Nashville Academy of Medicine hired its first executive secretary, Mr. Jack E. Ballentine, with a background in advertising and public relations. He came from Aladdin Industries, which he had helped to bring to Nashville when he worked for the Chamber of Commerce as industrial director. Academy members willingly paid an increase in dues to employ him.

The Academy promptly joined with the movement of organized medicine throughout the nation to heighten public appreciation of doctors after the recent scarring wars over costs, quackery, and indigent care. Under Dr. Hollis E. Johnson, its public service committee announced a far-reaching program committing doctors to new visibility and participation in Nashville life, while answering to the public demands for access to a doctor when most gravely needed, insurance against catastrophic illness, and a sufficient number of physicians for Tennessee.

These last included an emergency point of contact, putting everyone in touch with a doctor at anytime, day or night. The Academy also pledged to study legislation that would provide care for the family of a wage earner disabled for a long period of time. It promised to see whether a loan fund for medical students might be feasible. As to the cost issue, the Academy agreed to try to enroll every Davidson County physician in the state society's voluntary health insurance plan.

The entire public service program comprised eleven points; the other seven were public relations, including the creation of a grievance committee, essay contests for high school children who might be interested in medicine as a career, and more.

The Academy also took a stand in favor of a new consolidated city-county public hospital, which floundered in the miasma of local politics. It also called for fluoridated water and a solution to the inadequate sewerage system, terming it "the number one public health problem in the community." The agenda and minutes record numerous other initiatives, undertakings, and outreach activities, all meant to resist the Roosevelt and Truman administration national health insurance plans—but all intellectually honest endeavors to meet public wishes for more of the "old-timey doctor" of yore. Mr. Ballentine established a doctor's call service through the Academy phone lines, participated in all manner of meetings with friends like the Red Cross and Community Chest, set up medical exhibits and distributed literature at fairs and festivals—and much else.

In the early 1960s, the Academy set up quarterly meetings to which hospital staffs were invited. Dinner and a business session preceded scientific presentations, often given by department heads from hospitals outside Nashville. Societies of specialists continued to form as well. All the groups served the need of doctors for current information, so the proliferation of papers and presentations was not competitive but certainly required the busy practitioner to pick and choose among offerings.

NASHVILLE MEDICINE AND THE CIVIL RIGHTS MOVEMENT

In 1942 Dr. William A. Beck, professor of clinical medicine at Meharry, gave an address heard on radio around the nation. He cited the differential morbidity and mortality between white and black people from tuberculosis. "In the past thirty years," he told his listeners, "the mortality rate for the white race has been reduced from first to seventh place, whereas the mortality rate for the colored race has been reduced from first to second place." He called for a hearing at the "great bar of justice" for black sufferers, and he declared, "Absolutely no program for the control and eradication of tuberculosis can hope to be successful unless the opportunities for hospitalization and facilities for treatment are available equally to Negroes and to whites." That they were not equal was plain from statistics he cited from the National Tuberculosis Association. In the thirteen Southern states where two-thirds of the nation's Negro population lived, there had been 15,883 deaths in the most recent year's figures—but only 7,066 open to blacks.

Stopping short of demanding desegregation of tuberculosis and general hospitals, Dr. Beck let his statistics speak for themselves. Instead, he urged wider training opportunities for black doctors. Every community with a sizable black population needed a black physician who knew how to administer pneumothroax treatments, and every large city needed a black chest surgeon. (The entire South at that moment had not even one.) Black physicians required opportunity if they were to stop tuberculosis—"the Axis enemy here in America"—among their people.

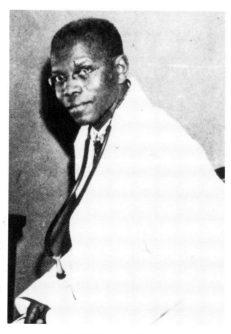

Dr. William A. Beck

Black Americans were more vulnerable to the most common health maladies than whites. In 1960 almost four times as many blacks died from tuberculosis as whites. The incidence of syphilis among blacks was roughly ten times greater on the basis of reported cases. The rate of black children dying from whooping cough, meningitis, measles, diphtheria, and scarlet fever was at least twice as high as that for white children. The rate of black mortality from cardiovascular disorders was about three times as high as the rate for whites. Black women who frequently bore most of the burden for earning a living in a black household were especially likely to fall victim to hypertensive heart disease. The deaths of black mothers in childbirth and of black babies in their infancy had been high over time, and such was still the case in the middle of the twentieth century. In 1959 complications arising out of pregnancy and childbirth resulted in maternal deaths among blacks four times as often as among whites. The death rate of black children before the age of one was almost two times as high as that of white children in the same group. Mental illness was another malady that occurred more frequently among blacks than among whites. In 1950 most of the patients in mental hospitals were blacks.

Aside from deleterious living conditions, one of the causes for the differential conditions in black and white health was racial discrimination in hospitals. If admitted—and some hospitals refused that—the black man or woman might have to wait for one of the few beds reserved for them, on a "colored ward" or floor. Blacks who sought treatment on an outpatient basis might or might not receive it. Some received humiliation for their pains. Such was the case of a black postal worker in Nashville who became ill on the job one day. From a roster of doctors approved by his federal employer—which included no black physician—he chose one, and upon arrival was made to sit in a broom closet.

Even the seriously ill black person who managed to find a hospital bed might be forced to give up his doctor if he or she too was black. To be appointed to the staff of a hospital or attend one's patients there, a physician had to belong to the local affiliate of the American Medical Association. Until the late 1940s most city and county medical societies refused to let black doctors join.

In 1946 the American Nurses Association opened membership to all qualified nurses, regardless of race, creed, or country of origin. It became the first professional organization in the United States to end racial discrimination in its ranks. The AMA followed suit in 1950, although more circumspectly. It merely instructed all chapters to "take such steps as they may elect" to eliminate membership restrictions based on race.

In the summer of 1954 the Giles County Medical Society opened its rolls to Drs. D. M. Spotwood and William A. Lewis, both graduates of Meharry Medical College. It did so, according to its public statement, "on the basis of education, training, experience, standing in the community, and the excellent job they are doing for our colored people." The two automatically became members of the Tennessee State Medical Association and the American Medical Association.

In September the Nashville Academy of Medicine amended its constitution and by-laws to make any qualified physician eligible for membership. In February, 1955, three members of the Meharry faculty—Drs. E. Perry Crump, Axel Hansen, and Matthew Walker—joined the organization.

Two months later, the outgoing president of the state medical association, Dr. John R. Thompson, told his colleagues:

> The profession as a whole has not faced up to problem and taken a definite lead in the solving of its perplexities. If an individual is qualified, he should be allowed to accept the privileges which go with that qualification, regardless of race, creed, or color of his skin. Courageous societies within our midst have taken this step. To them our congratulations.

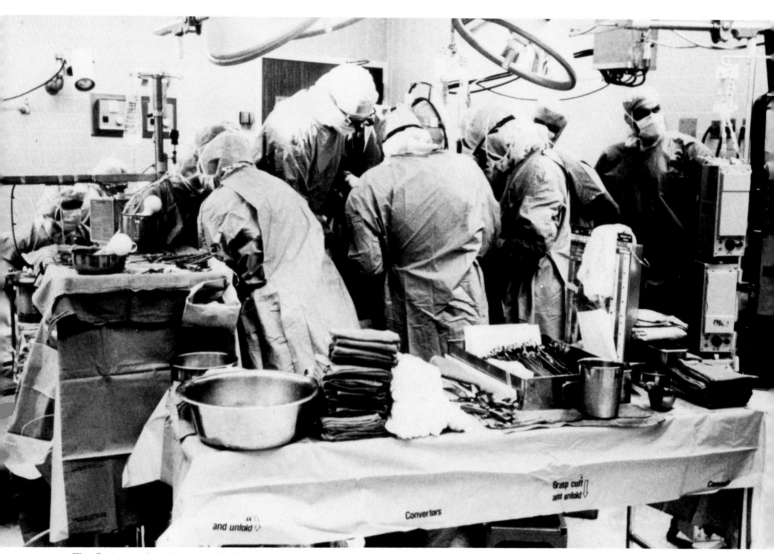

The first open-heart surgery in Tennessee, under a team headed by Dr. William Stoney, 1967, performed at St. Thomas Hospital.

Chapter Nine

THE NATION'S HEALTHCARE CAPITAL

By 1960 the profession in Nashville and Tennessee had succeeded in turning to account the burgeoning government presence, the threats against its state-guaranteed privileges, and public demand for more of its services at less cost.

Doctors worked out a *modus vivendi* with state and local health departments, accepting the enlarged government role in public health. It conceded the benefits of the measures enacted during the Progressive Era to assure pure food, milk, and water supplies. Governmental action against insect-borne disease, such as malaria, received a belated stamp of approval. Immunization, public education, and the relationship between the patient and his living environment remained a middle ground, with government and private physicians having a shared role.

Physicians also conceded that poor people needed adequate medical care, that the occasional grievance between a patient and a doctor might deserve adjustment, and that people who required medical care at nights and on an emergency basis ought to have it available.

Finally, the profession came to the consensus that every locale with a sizable population had to have a hospital and adequate diagnostic facilities. Thus the doctors at mid-century happily accepted the boon of federal dollars for hospital construction, notably the Hill-Burton Act and Veterans Administration measures. That these opened new opportunities for appointments, emoluments, and research were additional points in their favor. Organized medicine grew adept at lobbying the General Assembly; from the struggle over authority in the state health department and the routing of the naturopaths gave rise to the public affairs committees which monitored legislation and worked in liaison with counsel. From these roots, grew medicine's influential political action committees in later years.

THE COMING OF MEDICARE

Dr. Kyle Copenhaver, outgoing president of the state medical association took a remarkable stance in May, 1945. "I am convinced that we should make a realistic approach to finding a sensible middle course" between drastic federal intervention in medicine, and "our present system of practice." He called for a plan that would provide adequate medical care to everyone, especially the person of average means, since the rich could pay medicine's "pyramiding costs" and the poor could get services through government programs. Dr. Copenhaver proposed prepaid medical insurance for catastrophic illness, surgical, and hospital care, calling it "our only hope of defeating some form of government control."

Here was the essential, positive stance that organized medicine assumed in the postwar years. It could not prevail against government control only by arguing against "socialized medicine." Rather, doctors would have to take initiatives to solve the problems that the public complained of—high costs to all and prohibitive costs to the indigent, the shortage of doctors and hospitals in rural areas, the rising problem of chronic illness after the conquest of infectious disease, the need for round-the-clock availability of a doctor. In the words of Dr. Daugh W. Smith of Nashville:

> The people *don't want* socialized medicine, but they DO want something better than they have now. They want a more adequate voluntary health insurance program, with more doctors participating and less restricting clauses in the contract; they want a decent plan for the medically indigent; they want a fee schedule that does not vary from the sublime to the ridiculous; and they DEMAND a return to the sympathetic doctor-patient relationship.

To assure Tennesseans access to surgical and obstetrical care, the state association in 1949 established a voluntary health insurance plan. Insurance against the risk of illness was still new. Organized medicine first took an interest during the Depression, seeing such plans as a way to blunt the drive for national health insurance, but also to assist the many people with low or modest incomes now requiring a doctor's attention but with limited means to pay his fees. Some county medical societies set up service bureaus that organized patient bills and worked out their settlement on a prepayment or postpayment basis.

Voluntary prepayment plans gradually emerged as a popular choice, both by consumers and doctors. By 1950 nearly every state had a statewide plan in operation. Tennessee's state medical association began looking into prepayment insurance plans before the war, but implementation was delayed by the world crisis. In 1949, the association adopted a plan that provided for insurance to be written by private companies. In three years, 370,000 citizens obtained coverage. Under the "Tennessee Plan," participating physicians accepted from the insurance companies a schedule of fees as payment in full for all types of obstetrical and surgical services. To participate a family had to have an income no higher than $4,200, an individual no higher than $2,400. Other types of medical or health problems were not covered.

Although widely popular among physicians and the general public, the plan gradually became obsolete as postwar prosperity raised incomes for most families. Group health insurance as a fringe benefit spread in the workplace. Anticipating the world thirty years in the future, Dr. John R. Thompson observed, "Especially do [physicians] resent someone in the office of the insurance carrier setting their fee." The passage of Medicare made the pioneering Tennessee Plan finally obsolete, and the Association discontinued it, effective in 1967.

In 1953 the organized profession lent its support to a bill in the legislature that would assure free hospital and medical care for every indigent Tennessean. In Tennessee as throughout the nation, organized labor was the most powerful force in the cause of a health insurance system, be it contributory or compulsory.

Initially doctors strongly opposed the measure proposed in Congress by Aime Forand of Rhode Island, which would have provided hospital coverage for persons receiving Social Security payments. One person in six aged 65 and over entered a hospital each year, and hospital

Vanderbilt University Medical School

Faculty hoped that wartime stringencies and stress would be only "for the duration." Indeed, manpower returned to former levels, but the zeal and zest of the Thirties did not. The school lost some the faculty who had driven that energy, when Alfred Blalock departed for Hopkins, Tinsley Harrison moved on to

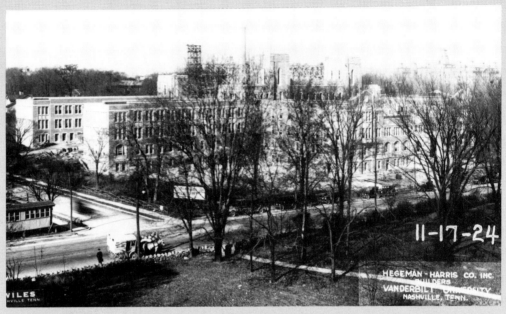

The new Vanderbilt University School of Medicine under construction, 1924

start medical departments elsewhere, and John Youmans accepted the deanship at the University of Illinois medical school.

The school was hard-hit by continuing deficits at the hospital, mainly because of empty beds and the costs of giving indigent care. The administration tried a proprietary approach: persuade more paying patients to come to Vanderbilt for hospital care. The second tack was to get the City of Nashville to pay for the care of poor people. A contract for this last was negotiated in 1949, but failed to solve the problem. When the city canceled the agreement, Vanderbilt offered to become Nashville's general hospital, but the City Council voted down the proposal.

The Vanderbilt Board of Trust finally separated the budgets of the ailing hospital and the robust medical school, and instructed the former's administrators to figure out how to pay its way, to get into the market for patients with personal funds, prepaid medical plans, or insurance. The hospital did some refurbishing of rooms and hallways, and also opened tertiary care facilities likely to draw persons with resources. The patients came, and by 1957 the hospital balanced its bottom line. Success was crowned with a $2.3 million grant from the Ford Foundation for a new "round wing."

In the late 1950s and early 1960s new subspecialties sprang up all along the corridors: allergies, pulmonary and cardiovascular diseases, nutrition, physiology and experimental medicine, endocrinology, gastroenterology, neurology. Surgery added new subspecialties, and former divisions of medicines became entirely new departments: ophthalmology, psychiatry, and others.

As early as 1946, a group of consultants told the administration that the medical school must become a "medical center," one committed to meeting the expectations of something called "the community"—for brighter quarters, humane treatment, and more magic bullets, like the sulfa drugs. The subsidies of the federal government, begun during the war emergency, continued, but the goal was now the purchase of those things that "the community" wanted: more beds, the latest equipment, 'space-age' facilities, more "health." All these

Some of the distinguished faculty of the Vanderbilt Medical School in the postwar years:

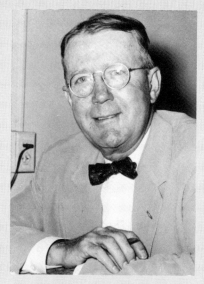

Dr. John Youmans, who served as dean from 1949 to 1958

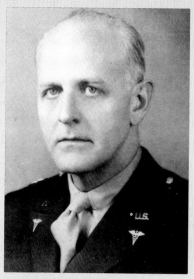

Dr. Hugh Morgan, wartime leader

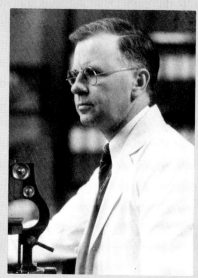

Dr. Ernest Goodpasture, once described by the Journal of the Tennessee Medical Association as "the greatest scientist produced in Tennessee"

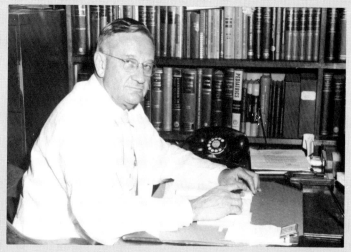

Dr. Rudolph Kampmeier, internist, scholar, historian

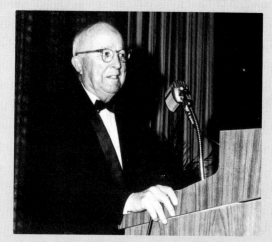

Dr. Frank Luton, psychiatrist

were to be regarded now like food, shelter, and clothing—as necessities of life—paid for by the recipient who could afford them, otherwise by insurance plans or by the government.

Washington also helped restore the school's once luminous stature as a center for productive medical research. Throughout the 1950s and 1960s, government grants for research grew, mostly for specific terms and specific projects.

Planning for the new medical center began in the mid-1960s, and in 1974 the Board of Trust projected a new hospital and medical education building. In 1977 the latter opened: Light Hall, built from funds from Dr. Rudolph A. Light and from the federal government. The new hospital completed in September, 1980, became the largest building Vanderbilt had ever erected.

The medical education program was big in all other ways, too. Between 1960 and 1980, the number of students doubled. Federal support to the school was in various ways conditioned on that growth in enrollment, which in turn required more facilities, which in turn required more grants, which in turn required more federal dollars . . . . In part because of a favorable ratio of teachers, Vanderbilt medical students received a great deal of individualized teaching, and they scored in or near the top of national measurements and rankings.

The hospital thrived on payment for services rendered. One faculty member observed that its patients were active "health care consumers" who have paid insurance that they could spend at the shiny pavilions of other institutions. Historian Timothy Jacobson has observed, "At Vanderbilt patient care, or service, is no longer an ancillary activity; it is a big business that increasingly fuels the whole enterprise."

An entirely new $40 million hospital opened in September, 1980. By mid-decade there was built around it a virtually new medical campus. A $6.5 million laser center and a $21.5 million research facility were dedicated in 1986. Two years later a $72 million outpatient department began serving the community, its halls and waiting rooms always crowded. Other renowned programs included a burn unit and a Children's Hospital. In 1986 Dr. Stanley Cohen won the Nobel Prize for Medicine, given for his work in cell growth factors. It was the second of this "greatest of earthly honors" to come to the school, Dr. Earl Sutherland having received the prize in 1971 for his contributions to understanding the mechanics of hormones.

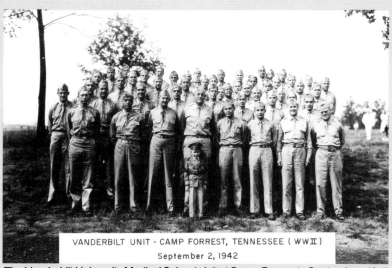

VANDERBILT UNIT - CAMP FORREST, TENNESSEE (WWII)
September 2, 1942

The Vanderbilt University Medical School Unit at Camp Forrest in September, 1942

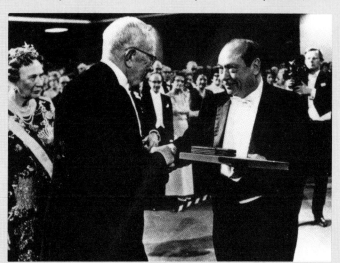

Dr. Earl Sutherland accepts the 1971 Nobel Prize in Medicine from the King of Sweden

Meharry Medical College

The six years of Dr. Edward L. Turner's administration (1938-1944) saw stronger emphasis on clinical instruction, the addition of specialized disciplines, and the first major support for faculty research. The nursing school won accreditation and began awarding the baccalaureate degree. The school of dentistry very nearly closed as applicants ebbed in the 1930s and new sources of support eluded officials. But with help from W. W. Kellogg, Turner appointed Dr. M. Don Clawson to undertake a reorganization of the school and by 1945, enrollment had been rebuilt. Clawson thus became a natural successor to Turner.

Not even the huge foundations could sustain Meharry forever, and in the postwar years President Clawson considered affiliating with the Southern Regional Compact. Part of the rationale behind the interstate plan was for Meharry to boost Meharry's enrollment and finances—but also to assure that other medical schools in the region could remain segregated. Alumni resoundingly opposed the idea. In 1952 they realized a dream long deferred when Dr. Harold D. West became Meharry's first black president. He presided over the college as the second American reconstruction swept over it and over Nashville.

As formerly all-white medical schools began to admit minority students, Meharry was compelled to reaffirm its mission and reason for existence. Dr. West guided the college through its own desegregation, and Meharry continued to receive powerful support from Washington in the years of the "Great Society," renewing the original mission of preparing clinicians and health care workers who would serve in poor and minority communities.

The presidential administration of psychiatrist Lloyd C. Elam saw a new physical plant built, including a new Hubbard Hospital, largely with dollars from Washington. Financial stability nonetheless eluded the institution, which began looking to federal "distress grants." In one year alone, 1978, some $17 million in tax dollars came to Meharry—but still it had eleven dollars of debt for every one in assets.

President David Satcher, who arrived in 1982, set out to build the endowment and staunch the flow of red ink. An early achievement was the dismissal of the $29 million federal debt owed for the construction of the hospital. A task force appointed by President Ronald Reagan recommended the cancellation, and Meharry held an official "mortgage burning" on February 1, 1983.

Dr. Satcher also took on the long-term issue of Meharry's care for Nashville's poor by pushing, and finally winning, a merger between Hubbard Hospital and Nashville General Hospital. With that task done, Meharry in 1992 launched a campaign for $101 million. Its academic and research programs still stressed health problems that struck with particular ferocity in poor and underserved populations of Americans. Having won the warm admiration of Nashville's political and economic elite, Dr. Satcher left in 1993 to accept an appointment in the Clinton Administration. In 1998 he was named Surgeon General of the United States.

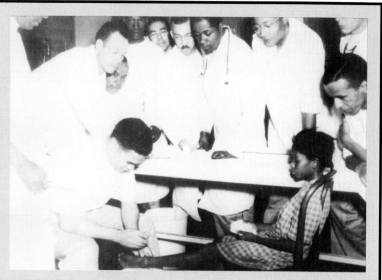

Orthopaedic clinic at Meharry in the 1940s

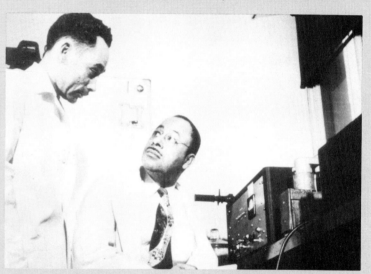

Dr. Harold D. West (seated) with Dr. Marion E. Zealey

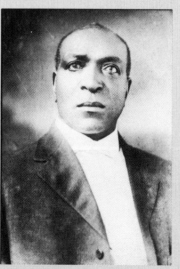

Dr. John Angelo Lester, physiologist and dean of Meharry Medical College

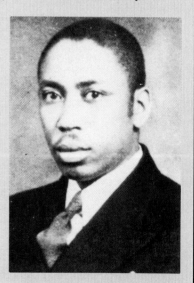

Dr. Matthew Walker, noted surgeon

care had doubled in price during the 1950s. As Dr. Charles Trabue noted, the proposal had a "very strong emotional appeal," and the contributory nature of Social Security blunted the accusation that it was state medicine on a piecemeal approach.

Popular response was powerful and favorable, and in 1960 Congress passed the Kerr-Mills Act, which provided federal funds for medicine programs for the aged poor. In Tennessee the program guaranteed for persons over 65, 15 days hospitalization, 90 days nursing home care, and certain essential drugs. The state medical association sent an informational mailing to Tennessee doctors and urged them to make the program effective, "since this is medicine's answer to the proposed government plan under the social security system for health care."

But most states simply failed to take advantage of Kerr-Mills; thus Medicare simmered on the agenda of the New Frontier. It lacked the votes to pass until after the Democratic sweep of 1964. The following year President Lyndon Johnson made it the first priority of his Great Society program. In final form, the law provided for compulsory hospital insurance under Social Security, government-subsidized voluntary insurance to cover physicians' bills, and expanded assistance to the states for medical care for the poor (Medicaid). President Johnson signed the programs into law on July 30, 1965.

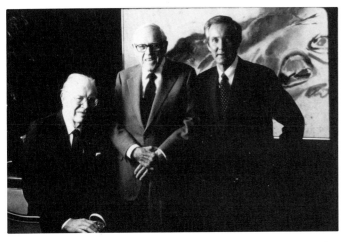

The founders of the Hospital Corporation of America. Left to right: Dr. Thomas Frist, Sr., Mr. Jack Massey, Dr. Thomas Frist, Jr.

The enactment of Medicare and Medicaid changed the face of American medicine. By the 1980s more than a third of all hospital costs were being paid by these federal insurance programs. These years saw the continued expansion of private health plans, as companies built worker benefit packages. Until very recent times a majority of people had paid for medical services at a hospital in cash. Now such institutions took in less than 10% of their revenues from this source.

THE RISE OF HOSPITAL CORPORATION OF AMERICA

Medicare had uniform standards for benefits, and it allowed physicians to charge above what the program would pay. With so many patients having their medical bills guaranteed, entrepreneurs saw a chance to operate hospitals for profit. The key was concentrating management over a chain of institutions and bringing about savings through such cost-saving business techniques as centralized purchasing, administration, accounting. In 1968, three important private hospital management groups entered the field, all based in Nashville.

Hospital Corporation of America actually began in frustration. Dr. Thomas Frist, Sr. and other physicians had bought Park View Hospital in 1956, and in the mid-1960s decided to sell it. They searched for a management company that would operate the facility and raise the capital to expand it. Looking around the nation, Dr. Frist found plenty of enterprises willing to acquire factories or banks, but none interested in hospitals. He called a meeting of his son, Dr. Thomas Frist, Jr., and Jack Massey, who had made a fortune in franchising Harlan Sanders' Kentucky Fried Chicken. Together the trio formed HCA, and in very few years it dominated the nation's hospital management business.

That same year, Nashville physicians Irwin Eskind and Herbert Schulman formed Hospital Affiliates International, calling on the business acumen of Baron Coleman and Richard Eskind. General Care Corporation started in

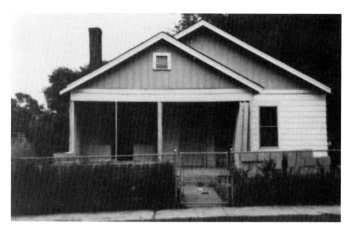

The first headquarters of HCA, September, 1968.

1968 as well, remaining small relative to its two giant competitors.

HCA and HAI, publicly traded securities companies, bought old hospitals, built new ones, and managed others under contract. HCA's Nashville institutions included Donelson, Hendersonville, Southern Hills, Edgefield, and West Side, as well as the flagship Park View.

By 1980 HCA owned or managed 140 hospitals. That decade forced hard decisions on the company, however, as Washington lowered the ceiling on costs of procedures for Medicare patients. HCA also overreached itself, acquiring the rival Hospital Affiliates International and trying but failing to take control of the American Hospital Supply Corporation. The popular press was only too happy to print stories that suggested the company was more interested in profits than people.

Attempting to recoup its position, HCA sold 140 acute care facilities it owned to another local firm, HealthTrust, run by former HCA executives. Its vast holdings still included more than 80 general hospitals and 53 psychiatric hospitals. It managed 200 others under contract. In 1988 the firm went private and was sold for $4.5 billion to a group of private investors headed by Dr. Thomas Frist, Jr. "Doctors can certainly enjoy a good living," he once mused to a reporter, "but I don't know many who accumulate tremendous wealth. You must do it outside the practice of medicine." When he became head of the new HCA, the 51-year-old physician had never practiced his profession except for a two-year stint as an Air Force flight surgeon.

HCA went public again in 1992, a $700 million deal. With facilities in Europe and Latin America, the company spanned the planet. Then a week after the Clinton Administration proposed its plan to reform the nation's health care system, Dr. Frist announced a merger with Louisville's Columbia Health Care Corporation and the prospect of a move to that city.

After Columbia / HCA accused Kentucky officials of reneging on promises to repeal a state tax on hospitals—and Nashville offered a huge tax break—chief executive Richard Scott announced that his company would relocate to Nashville. At the same time, it planned a merger with HCA spinoff, HealthTrust. When that was complete,

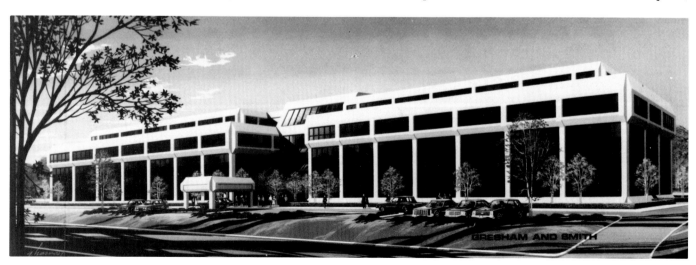

In 1981, the company opened its new corporate headquarters.

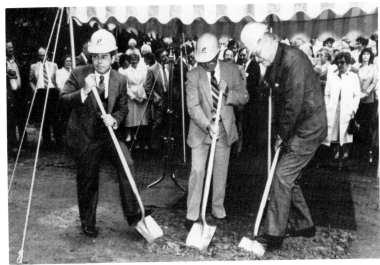
Dr. Frist, Sr., right, helps break ground for a new HCA facility.

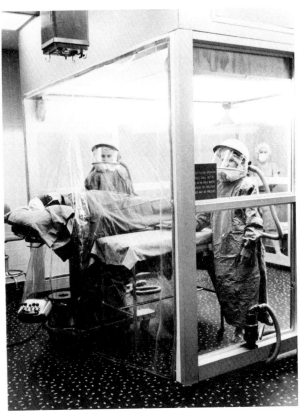
Baptist Hospital's first total hip replacement, 1971. The surgery was performed in this super-sterile "greenhouse."

Columbia / HCA owned 199 hospitals and 128 outpatient clinics in 34 states, England, and Switzerland, and South America, with annual revenue of $15 billion. Having 23 hospitals in Tennessee, it was by far the state's largest corporation.

Columbia / HCA faced its time of troubles. In March, 1997, federal agents began raiding its hospitals with search warrants and accusing the vast company of systematically scheming to defraud Government health insurance programs. In July Richard Scott resigned as chief executive officer and was replaced by Dr. Frist, Jr. New faces were put in place across top levels of management. Three Columbia executives in Florida, the epicenter of the scandal, were indicted, and analysts speculated whether the giant, now on its knees, was mortally wounded.

The new managers abandoned the company's obsession with growth and promised a kinder, gentler corporate face. Dr. Frist put the home care division up for sale and pledged to compress the chain by selling at least a third of its hospitals.

His father, Dr. Frist, Sr., evidently felt Columbia had strayed and was saddened by the fraud investigation. On his death on January 4, 1998, Dr. Frist was warmly remembered for his part in developing the city into the nation's health care capital, with its eighteen publicly-traded healthcare companies and more than one hundred private ones.

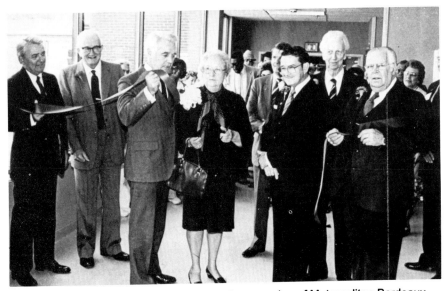
Nashville Mayor Richard Fulton opens the new wing of Metropolitan Bordeaux Hospital, named for Dr. Lenor de Sa Ribeiro, third from right, in 1983

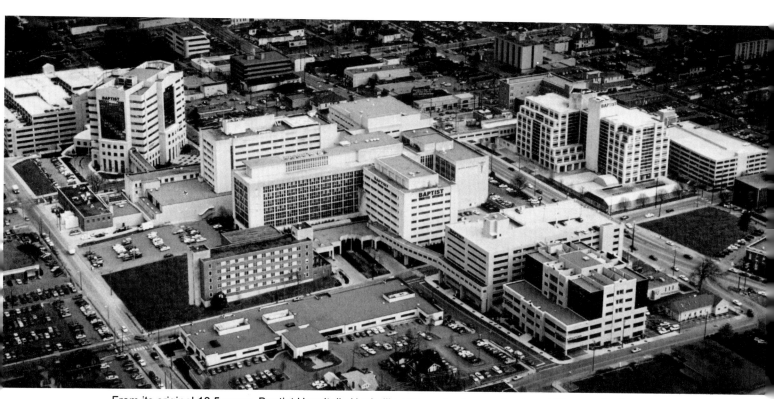

From its original 10.5 acres, Baptist Hospital's Nashville campus had grown to almost 38 acres by the mid-1990s.

Chapter Ten

A NEW CENTURY OPENS

---

*I*n Nashville and throughout the nation, the federal government also invested vast sums in hospital building after World War II. Money from Washington had subsidized the wartime industries, then helped build the urban renewal projects around town. The city welcomed more of this largess for health. The Veterans Administration Hospital was one such project. The Hill-Burton Act of 1946 provided funds to build in areas of the country lacking them. Ten years later more than 50 facilities had been completed and were in operation, supplying some 2,400 beds. By 1962, Tennessee was one of the leading states in the South in number of hospital beds per population. With 8.1 beds per thousand people, the state exceeded the national average of 7.5 per thousand. In Nashville Hubbard Hospital and Vanderbilt Hospital expanded their facilities with Hill-Burton funds. Funds under the law also assisted in construction of the John J. Lentz Public Health Center, which opened in 1960, and Nashville Memorial, opening in 1965.

The burgeoning medical schools, teaching hospitals, and ancillary institutions, along with their executive and administrators, constituted a new system that counterbalanced doctors in private practice. Institutional medicine had its own interests and sought a role for itself in and a share of any public program. Some effort to bring order to this growth was begun in 1964 with the founding of the Nashville Metropolitan Region Health and Hospital Planning Council. The Nashville Area Chamber of Commerce saw the need for such an agency to eliminate waste and duplication of services. An independent organization operating under a state charter, the Council surveyed existing hospital and health care facilities and made recommendations for expansion of these or construction of new ones. Dr. Charles C. Trabue, IV, served as first president of the council, which included other business and civic leaders.

THE SECOND GREAT AGE OF HOSPITAL-BUILDING

Nashville's second great age of hospital building began in this period and continued into the 1990s. HCA built its first hospital, Donelson Hospital, in 1970 to serve a rapidly growing section of Davidson County. Miller Clinic announced

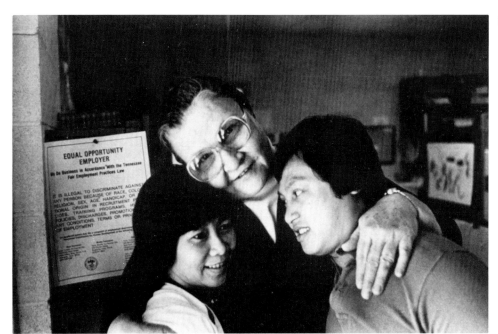

Sister Andrea Vaughan shares a hug with two friends at St. Thomas Hospital

a $2.5 million expansion in the late summer of 1971. Ground was broken for the new St. Thomas Hospital on Harding Road in April, 1972. The next month Madison Hospital officials rolled out plans for an additional 92 beds. Another new facility, West Side Hospital, opened that fall.

In the same period, Nashville General began a new Children's Clinic and remodeled clinics for tumor and heart treatment and oral and ear-nose-throat surgery. Hubbard Hospital started construction of a new hospital, which was dedicated at the centenary of Meharry Medical College in 1976. Madison Hospital added a new wing with almost 100 beds. Parthenon Pavilion, a psychiatric hospital that was part of HCA's Park View complex, made plans for 50 more beds. Vanderbilt opened its new fetal care unit, overseen by Dr. Mildred Stahlman. The State of Tennessee announced new facilities at Central State Hospital, including a drug and alcohol treatment center and a children and youth program. Financial equilibrium in hospitals proved intensely cyclical and with the recession of the early 1980s a number of Nashville institutions were advertising in an effort to fill empty beds and vying for special populations, like birthing mothers. Nonetheless, in 1983 the city's hospitals projected $60 million in expansions.

That was dwarfed by the stupendous growth starting up a decade later. In 1992 six more major hospital construction projects were underway or on the drawing board:

- **Baptist Hospital:** a $35.6 million, nine-story patient tower and $14 million office building and parking garage
- **Centennial Medical Center:** a $130 million, eight-story patient tower and office building
- **Donelson Hospital:** a $40-50 million replacement and five-story medical building. Named Summit Medical Center, it opened in December, 1994
- **St. Thomas Hospital:** seeking approval of government facilities needs panels for a $54.8 million expansion
- **Southern Hills Medical Center:** a $26 million expansion
- **Vanderbilt Medical Center:** an $80 million, 11-story patient tower

The most important hospital story of the 1990s was the Metropolitan Government's decision to merge Nashville General and Hubbard Hospital of Meharry Medical College. The idea had first been proposed about 1948, in the age of segregation, but required the sagacity of Dr. David Satcher, the will of Mayor Philip Bredesen, and an en-

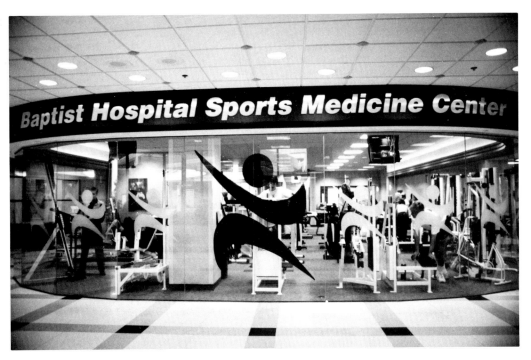

tirely different time. Critics who said General's old clientele would never accept hospitalization at Meharry were proved wrong. For its part, Meharry had to cope with operating its hospital under government rules, never easy, and to win back the middle-class black clientele it had sought, who were not sure they wanted to be treated in a hospital that had served poor people so well for so long.

THE ONGOING 'CRISIS'

Nashville's growth in hospitals came at a moment when politicians and the popular press discovered a "crisis" in the nation's health care system. Costs were rising like a rocket, so it was generally held. The deeper indictment held that Americans were not getting their money's worth. Reporters and editorial writers who took the crisis as their subject almost invariably observed that the United States had higher infant mortality rates and lower life expectancy than most European nations.

In the postwar years organized medicine had preserved doctors' privileges and standing that had been so hard won. They stood the ground that the sanitarians had taken, in the late nineteenth century until science gave physicians a powerful armamentarium of useful and workable therapies. Preventive medicine was a medicine that worked; and so gave doctors in the Nashville Academy of Medicine and the state medical association authority to ask for control over their own profession. This the state granted them, but for the next century the relations between government and medicine were perplexed and conflicted.

A medicine that worked—medicine based in science—joined food, clothing, and shelter as a necessity of life, in the public mind. Franklin D. Roosevelt's New Deal took up the clarion call of progressivism, which included an active role by government in the protection of maternal and child health, and the resistance to preventable problems of morbidity and mortality like tuberculosis and venereal disease. Public health, medicine's original great modern triumph, became formerly organized into government bureaucracies and thus, medicine became a service.

But these twin ideals—science and service—made at best an uneasy alliance. The public wanted ever more of medicine's services, and in the postwar decades many came to regard health care as a right that government should guarantee. Physicians who had never turned away a patient who could not pay nonetheless resented and

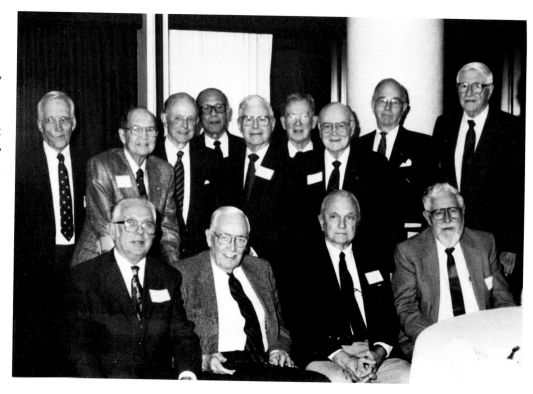

Thirteen physicians receive pins from the Nashville Academy of Medicine recognizing each one's fifty years of practice in medicine, 1994. Front row left to right: Drs. Paul Crane, Clarence Woodcock, Douglas Riddell, Russell Ward. Back row, left to right: Drs. Lindsay Bishop, Frank Witherspoon, David Pickens, Axel Hansen, Rowe Driver, Roy Parker, John Thomison, John Beveridge, Glenn Hammonds.

resisted law and regulation that impinged on their perogatives.

For all its achievements, medicine's resources were not infinite, even if popular expectation was. Who would receive which of its benefits was bound to be allocated. If the government proposed to do that, physicians objected. When politicians called for a marketplace solution, their fax machines jammed with letters from interest groups demanding fairness. The result ,in the last quarter of the century, was typically American: compromises that assured everybody something.

The "public service" drive of organized medicine had quelled the call for national health insurance in the 1940s. In the late 1960s it was sounded again, again by organized labor. Officials of the AFL-CIO and others proposed various national health insurance plans, each providing basic coverage for every citizen guaranteed by the federal government. Even the AMA put forward its own national health insurance proposal. For a time enactment by Congress of one or another of them seemed inevitable. As the Nixon Administration quailed before the rapidly rising costs of Medicare and Medicaid, it appeared that this

conservative President might sign such a bill into law.

Everything had inflated costs, and sick people felt it. The therapeutic advances of the prewar years had been mainly due to pharmacology, and drugs were cheap to produce. After 1960 gains came through expensive machines and costly procedures. Doctors needed more and better trained assistants to manage these new tools and techniques. The same employees demanded, fairly, that their wages be made comparable to those in other industries. When doctors discovered that Medicare and Medicaid would pay their "usual and customary fees"—i.e., whatever they billed—their charges increased. Seeing a patient in the hospital, one could bill more than seeing the same patient in one's office.

Patients wanted more services, the doctor earned more from an increase in the number and complexity of procedures. Insurance companies profits rose with the total volume of expenditures. Hospital costs spiraled upward. Everyone won—except people who had no insurance, employers who paid for group plans, and everyone who paid the taxes that financed Medicare and Medicaid.

These last two were natural political allies of the Nixon

Administration. In February, 1974, the President pronounced national health insurance "an idea whose time has come in America." His plan covered every citizen, using private insurance companies to provide coverage for workers and a separate government-run program for everyone else. Patients would pay 25% of medical bills, up to $5,000 a year.

If Watergate had not brought down the administration that summer, the nation might have had such a program. None again had a serious chance for adoption for another twenty years.

THE BY-WORD: COST CONTAINMENT

In a public statement in 1977, the Nashville Academy of Medicine queried whether Medicare and Medicaid repaid the physician what he or she actually spent to treat patients. More outpatient services should be covered by private insurers, it insisted, and physicians ought to sit on the decision-making bodies of all governmental planning agencies. Of them, there seemed no end.

At the same time, it urged its members to help contain health-care costs. Doctors should talk to their patients about bills, payments, and obligations, said a circular letter. All physicians ought to become "cost conscious and exercise discretion consistent with good medical care in determining the necessity for specific procedures, tests., and ancillary services." While criticizing, with some justification, the incapacity of government-sponsored health programs, medicine now stood in a defensive posture on the problem that so many feared, an inability to afford the price of seeing a doctor, should the need arise.

The 1980s saw the rising popularity of health maintenance organizations, providing medical care at lower expense mainly by reducing hospital admissions. HMOs were not a full and final answer to burgeoning costs of health care. In one year alone—1987 to 1988—the average daily charge for a hospital stay in Nashville increased by 11%. Persons without insurance—and that population included many young mothers with sick youngsters—

often found doors closed. By 1991 a day's stay in a hospital in Tennessee cost $1,233 on the average, and in the next year charges rose by more than 17%.

"Health care costs at a crisis state," read a headline in the *Tennessean* in the summer of 1992. It was old news, but in an election year candidates once again brought the matter to the public agenda. Organized medicine responded with something like hysteria. "We are now poised on the brink of a health care system breakdown," said Dr. George Lundberg, editor of the AMA's *Journal.* "In a worse-case scenario Congress would panic and nationalize the entire health-care industry."

True enough, 35 million Americans lacked health insurance, and the collapse of an over-extended economy was forcing a record number of personal bankruptcies. The driving force behind the new alarm may have been the demand by employers, beginning in the mid-1980s, that their workers pay a larger share of their health plans. Out-of-pocket spending paid by the patient slipped from 56% of all health care costs to about 20% in 1992. The government or private insurers picked up the difference. As the medical system spent thirteen cents of every dollar of goods and services produced in the country—up from five cents in 1960—both of those parties decided they could not afford it any longer.

The Clinton Administration's "Health Security Act," introduced in Congress in September, 1993, proposed permanent health insurance coverage for all Americans; required employers to pay for at least eighty percent of the cost of a basic package of benefits; placed every citizen into new quasi-governmental health care alliances to increase their leverage with insurers and providers; and capped the annual increase in health insurance premiums. The 1,342 page bill touched every problem area of the health care system, from workers compensation to the shortage of primary care physicians.

As with the national health insurance proposals of the early 1970s, passage of the plan seemed inevitable at first. But a year after its introduction, U. S. Senate Majority

Leader George Mitchell declared the plan dead. Big business, originally a supporter, became convinced that the proposal would mean new taxes and more regulation from Washington about the kind of insurance they would have to provide. Small business groups worried that the costs would force them to lay off workers.

That message was widely heard and believed. So was the Health Insurance Association's famous "Harry and Louise" commercials, featuring a yuppie couple pulling out technical-sounding provisions that, according to the ads, meant that Americans would pay more for less coverage.

TennCare Takes the Field

Closer to home, the State of Tennessee in January 1994 began TennCare. This managed care system provided coverage to about 1.2 million people, nearly one-quarter of the state's entire population. This included 750,000 Medicaid patients and an additional 400,000 people who were previously uninsured. It was a generous program, but the dollars were tight, and the incentive was with the managed care organizations to cut costs of care drastically.

TennCare arose out of an alarming situation. In 1993 Governor Ned McWherter saw that Medicaid costs had ballooned from 13.4% of the state's budget in 1987 to more than 26%. He presented the General Assembly with a managed care program crafted by his commissioner of finance and administration, David Manning. The legislation was embodied in a bill only one-and-one-half pages long. It passed with virtually no debate.

The transition from a fee-for-service system to the new system, wherein the state contracted with twelve privately-run managed care organizations, was chaotic. Many patients did not know which managed care group they belonged to, and it could take hours to get through to TennCare's phone lines. The managed care organizations were sometimes four or five months in reimbursing providers, who were already unhappy with TennCare's lower fee schedules.

One of TennCare's undoubted successes was bringing Medicaid patients into the mainstream and an end to the so-called "Medicaid mills." But this was accomplished with cunning if not virtual coercion. A physician who opted out of TennCare was not permitted to participate in BlueCross and BlueShield's commercial network, thereby losing a huge amount of potential business from 1.2 million people not on Medicaid. Still, almost one-third of doctors in BlueCross and BlueShield at first refused to join TennCare. Most later signed on.

People who never had health care coverage were "happy just to have a TennCare card in their pockets," said Gordon Bonnyman, a Nashville legal services lawyer. But critics claimed that the worse a patient's problems, the worse the system worked. Profits for the managed care groups depended on attracting healthy members who required little or no treatment in a given year. Penny-pinching administrators often vetoed doctors' decisions if they meant big outlays.

Many doctors felt that the budget for taking care of poor Tennesseans was balanced on their backs. According to a GAO report comparing TennCare's reimbursement rates with old Medicaid levels, doctors received slightly higher fees for visits and consultations, but for some forms of treatment they received 20% to 50% less than they did before. Said Dr. Winston Griner, "The poor are sicker. They consume more responsibility of my time and my colleagues' time, the hospitals' time, the home health agencies' time. They require more pharmaceutical support, more devices to support their needs and maintain and restore health. Those patients are making up 45 to 50 percent of our visits, but they provide only 17 percent of our revenues."

The failure of the Health Security Act left the field to TennCare and like plans around the country. Advocates contended that the managed-care organizations assured high-quality health care while containing costs. Critics charged that physicians were given financial incentives to limit tests, resulting in inaccurate diagnoses and inadequate treatments.

Managed care was essentially a new system of medicine, and another typically American compromise: regulated enterprise. Only the regulators were not the government, as organized physicians had long feared, but private, for-profit industry. For most of the century, making services available to poor people had perplexed lawmakers and physicians, and as the year 2000 approached, the problem was not solved. Managed care seemed likely to become an issue in the first national biennial elections of the new century.

Meanwhile, Nashville physicians took the new system in stride, for the most part. "There was a time when we decided what to charge," observed Dr. James O. Miller, a Madison obstetrician. "Now we accept what someone says we've earned." He had delivered 3,000 babies at the time, and he intended to go on doing so until it was time to retire.

COMPETITION RETURNS

If the state presence in medicine was fraught with difficulty, many doctors who had come into the profession in midcentury looked askance on the market revolution. In 1978 the advertisements by individual Nashville physicians appeared for the first time in the modern era. Although initially halted by court rulings, the ban was overturned, and doctors' ads became commonplace. By the 1990s, Nashville doctors' ads spread thickly through the midsection of the telephone company's Yellow Pages, beamed down from billboards, wrapped around city buses. Perhaps the most aggressive promoters of medical goods and services were the city's hospitals. Each one had a marketing department; the largest ones retained sophisticated and expensive public relations counsel. Not unlike the self-promoting doctor complained of by the *Nashville Journal of Medicine and Surgery* so long ago, they unabashedly sought "newspaper renown." The traditionalists in the profession objected, but the wheel was revolving again as many doctors repossessed the entrepreneurial view of their practices that an earlier generation had had.

These years saw the rise of new specialties like sports medicine, and the coming of 'round-the-clock streetcorner clinics and minor emergency medical centers. Dr. Karen Duffy, who owned one of the early ones in Nashville, observed that they quickly integrated into the overall health care system.

Joint replacement, major organ transplants, and cardiac pacemakers were greeted with fanfare in the early 1970s, to become commonplace thereafter. New techniques in non-invasive surgery, the CAT scanner, and magnetic resonance imaging arrived in Nashville in the early 1980s, followed in a few years by bone marrow transplants and arthroscopic surgery. The new technology undoubtedly contributed to the rise in the costs of health care, accounting for perhaps a third of it. Dr. John Lamb offered another view of the matter when he said, "In my opinion, it is totally forgotten by those who say medical costs are out of control that we can do things previously impossible in the history of mankind."

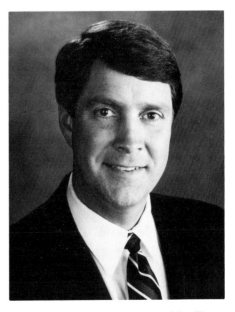

Dr. William H. Frist, youngest child of Dr. Thomas F. Frist, Sr. and Dorothy Cate Frist, transplant surgeon, and United States Senator

SIGNS OF THE TIMES

By the mid-1980s, homeless people had become a common sight on the streets of the city. This was not the population to whom hospital marketing campaigns were aimed. As glittering new towers rose on Murphy Avenue and in Antioch and Madison, Nashville's ill and indigent people relied as ever on dowdy old Nashville General for help from frostbite, anemia, or chest pains. An occasional physician also took to the street, to do what could be done; professor emeritus of pathology John Shapiro of Vanderbilt was one of them.

In the winter of 1989, surgeon Harold C. Dennison, Jr. died of complications from AIDS, thought to have been contracted in the care of a patient. Surgeons became wary and watchful, and the Nashville Academy of Medicine suggested that patients be tested where the chance of transmissibility existed.

The women's movement touched obstetricians and gynecologists, who sometimes saw evidence of spousal abuse. The practice of midwifery gained some adherence, and some practitioners, in the late years of the century, partly in response to feminists' assertion that such a critical life event could be "demedicalized" and removed from the hospital to the home, where it had once routinely happened.

Debate continued over the alleged doctor shortage in Tennessee. Studies essentially showed that the big cities were adequately supplied with physicians but rural counties strained for essential services like prenatal and obstetrical care. A like situation prevailed around the nation. Nashville's representative in the U. S. House, Clifford Allen, called for a national medical school to address the problem. Tennessee opened its fourth such institution, at East Tennessee State University. Once again the Volun-

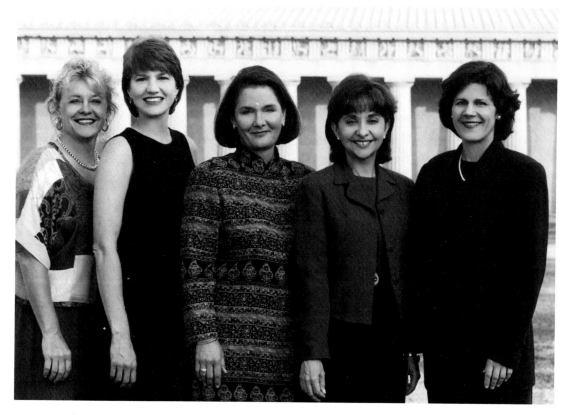

The present and past presidents of Tennessee Women in Medicine. Left to right: Dr. Lois W. Agstrom (1992-93), plastic surgery; Dr. Jennifer Oakley (1994-95), obstetrics and gynecology; Dr. Jill Chambers (1996), obstetrics and gynecology; Dr. Deborah German (1997), rheumotology; Dr. Maria Frexes-Steed (1998), general surgery

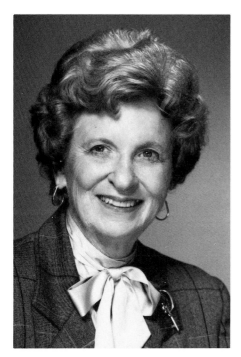

Dr. Sarah H. Sell, who in 1987 became the first woman to serve as president of the Nashville Academy of Medicine

teer State was doing its part in training more doctors for wherever they were needed.

Although effective political organization had preserved doctors' autonomy against actual government control, individual physicians felt the increased burden of regulation. They also paid dearly for insurance against malpractice as some juries found for plaintiffs and awarded ruinous penalties. Dr. John Thomison, Academy president, lamented that trial lawyers made physicians prey. To aid doctors to obtain coverage at affordable rates, the Tennessee Medical Association set up the State Volunteer Mutual Insurance Company.

Beginning in the late 1970s the popular press turned a relentless gaze on doctors accused of illegally prescribing drugs or making actionable misjudgments in patient care. Physicians accused in these cases sometimes received harsh publicity that destroyed their careers.

Local doctors were also called before the state licensure board because they had stopped life support for patients who were irreversibly comatose. Still others were picketed by anti-abortionists. In this period, medical ethics

became a serious discipline and concern in the health sciences.

Not all the legal action was in one direction, however. A noted plastic surgeon had to threaten to take the husband of a patient to court; it seems he refused to settle her bill for a popular kind of elective cosmetic surgery once he viewed the result.

AT ITS CENTENARY, A LEADERSHIP ROLE

In the early 1970s, the Nashville Academy of Medicine renewed its commitment to involvement in issues of public concern by undertaking disaster planning for the city and enlisting in a campaign against drug abuse. The origin for the former initiative is obscure, although Nashville had come close to serious civic disorder in a civil rights protest in 1967, and other cities had seen large-scale rioting. Addiction was clearly a growing wrong: in 1971 the city had some 1,000 hard-core drug users who lived to serve their habit. About one of every 100 Nashvillians between 18 and 35 had a drug-related problem. The Academy warned its members that dispensing drugs to

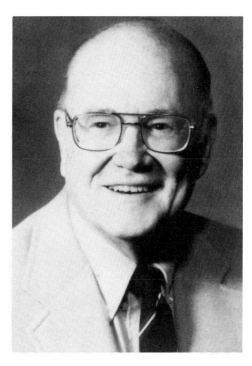

Dr. John Thomison. At the centennial year of the Nashville Academy of Medicine, Dr. Thomison called a unified profession to resist the "bureaucrats at various levels . . . , the trial lawyers . . . , and all those who would control us."

addicts, outside of court-sponsored programs, was a crime, and urged them to restrain prescribing amphetamines, a lawful drug being widely abused.

Staff recruited members to contribute their time as team doctors for senior high sports, and many responded. They stood in a tradition, whether they knew it or not; some Nashville doctors of the '90s, including Tom Tompkins of Tennessee Orthopaedic Alliance, look back on the physicians who took care of their injuries on the playing field as their first inspiration to study medicine. It was the beginning of a focus on sports medicine for the city's amateur and professional athletes, which by the late 1990s had become a major emphasis of some practices and dedicated services at area hospitals.

Other doctors went on the air, on a monthly radio program broadcast started by WLAC in 1963, to discuss health matters. A local television station featured physicians in "Town Meetings," discussing issues made popular by the lay press such as nutrition, the risks of fatty foods, and the importance of exercise. The program was eventually picked up by the midstate affiliate of the public broadcasting service, WDCN.

The Academy's most popular public service activity was "Tel-Med," begun in January, 1975. This nationwide program provided three-to-five minute tape recordings, available by telephone, about health concerns and problems. Family health guides and reference books written for lay people sold well. The proprietors behind Tel-Med provided the information for a post-literate society, and distributed it under sponsorship of local medical societies. In its first two weeks of operation, Tel-Med received almost 11,000 calls, and the number kept climbing.

In the nation's bicentennial year, 1976, the Academy's sixteen standing and special committees comprised 150 of its members. The panels put on their agendas a wide range of scientific, economic, political, and public service questions. That same summer the board began recruiting members to supervise mass immunizations against swine flu, a widely feared catastrophe that never materialized. Across the nation another supposed prevalent health problem, "child abuse," seized the public attention, and in May, 1977, the Academy focused a program on that subject. In later years, Nashville and Tennessee physicians enlisted in the fight against the spread of HIV (human immunodeficiency virus) infection, and to provide health, social, and support service for those infected by it.

The Academy's board and officers continued to take the lead on vital issues. It commented on local and state health initiatives it considered deleterious to public welfare, and it urged positive changes for the general well-being of Nashville. When physicians lambasted the proposal of Mayor Bill Boner

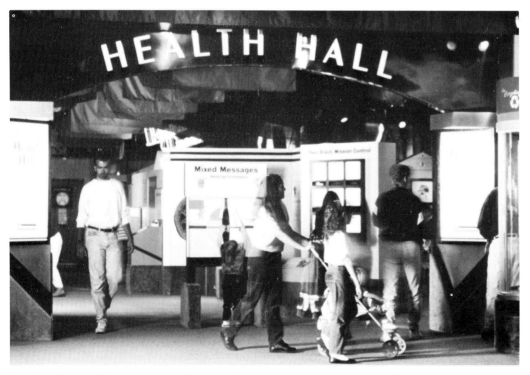

The Health Hall at the Cumberland Science Museum, a project of the Nashville Academy of Medicine

for a "landfill" (i.e., garbage dump) sited near the Cumberland River, they had come full circle. A century earlier their predecessors had made Nashville's public health a particular concern, and won significant support for medicine's most effective regimen, prevention. A Health Hall, which the Academy sponsored at the Cumberland Science Museum, reminded visitors that Nashville was about health care as well as the health business.

Doctors of Nashville in the year 2000 recognize those of 1800 only by ties of sentiment, for they have little common understanding. Since that time—not so very long ago—knowledge of the complexity of human biology has multiplied beyond the telling. Yet the history of medicine remains an important ancillary branch of this new scientific and technical base. As Dr. J. T. Moore of Tennessee wrote in 1952, "We have gathered the choice grain from the work and inventive genius of all medical men of many centuries past."

Dr. Charles Beck, of Madison, once noted that one of his reasons for choosing medicine as his profession was that one could never learn everything, yet could learn something new every day. So it is with history, and the history of medicine in Nashville.

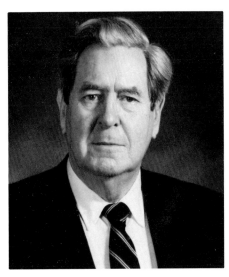

Nashville surgeon Benjamin F. Byrd, Jr. served as president of the American Cancer Society in 1975-1976, one of many Nashville physicians to head national medical and health organizations.

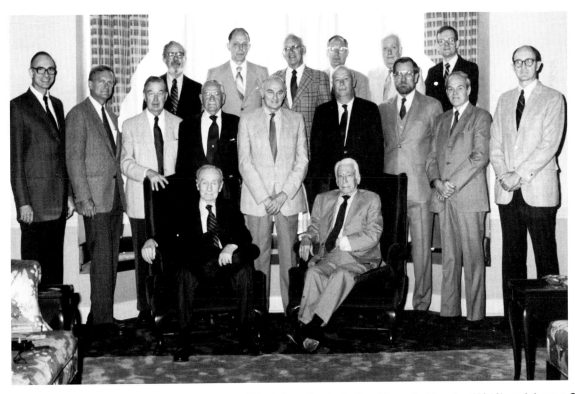

Some of the past presidents of the Nashville Academy of Medicine. Seated: Drs. Henry L. Douglas (1943) and James C. Gardner (1956). First row: Drs. Charles M. Hamilton (1979), Paul R. Stumb, III (1983), Joseph M. Ivie (1962), Rudolph H. Kampmeier (1951), William G. Kennon, Jr. (1958), William F. Meacham (1966), James W. Hays (1977), George W. Holcomb, Jr. (1974), Robert W. Ikard (1981), Back row: Louis Rosenfeld (1969), David R. Pickens, Jr. (1974), Addison B. Scoville, Jr. (1964), Frank W. Womack, Jr. (1973), Robert L. McCracken (1971), Ronald E. Overfield (1982)

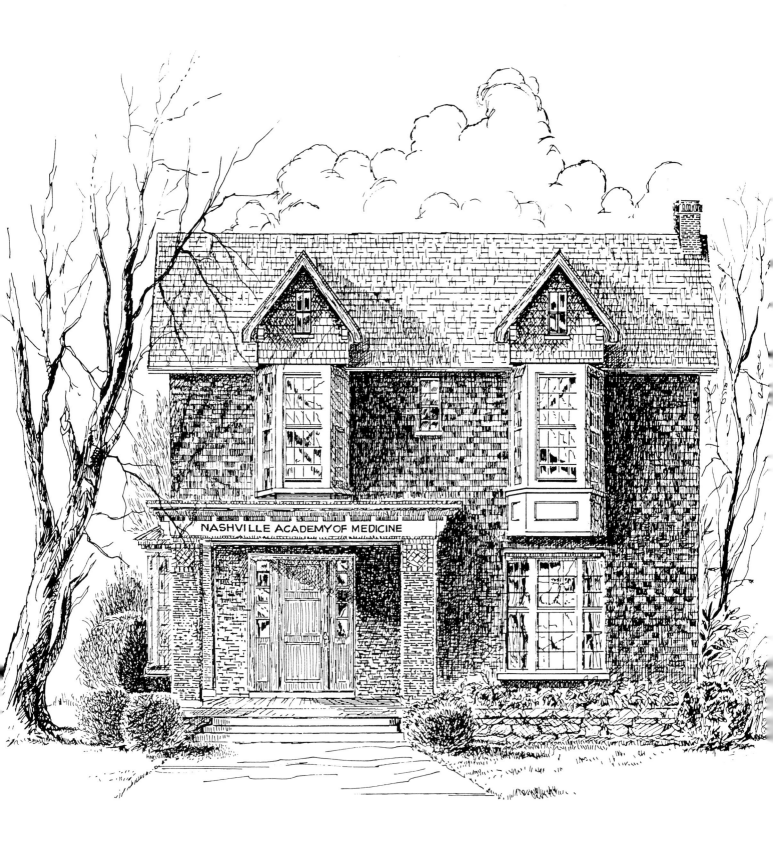

PROFILES IN NASHVILLE MEDICINE

Nashville's physicians love their work. When asking if they found satisfaction in the labor they do, one might expect to find a bell-curve distribution; not so. An interviewer who compiled the pages that follow recalled the enthusiasm for the practice of medicine that the doctors conveyed to him. "I just love these old lumbar problems that my patients present to me!" one orthopaedic surgeon exclaimed. Another doctor who cares for very sick newborn babies remarked, "We could not do this work if we were not passionate about it."

Another common, although not universal, characteristic among this group of physicians was their discovery of a direction toward medicine early in life. Some had been exposed to the work by parents or other relatives who were physicians. Others learned early that they had an interest and aptitude in science as well as a deep curiosity about how living things work. Among those interviewed for these pages, it was the rare physician who had not settled on medicine as a career before undergraduate school.

Many of the doctors interviewed for this book recalled one or more special teachers. An instructor might be remembered because he had provided an example of scientific erudition combined with kindness and compassion toward patients. Other doctors recalled their teachers who "made me think, not just regurgitate facts" or "showed me how to reason through problems."

Finally, the interviewer remembers with gratitude the graciousness with which he was received by busy physicians and their office or clinical staffs. With their phones ringing and their fax machines purring, virtually all gave him their time as if they had nothing more urgent to do. That impersonal kindness is another hallmark of Nashville medicine.

The physicians and institutions featured on the following pages have generously contributed to make possible the publication of Nashville Medicine: A History. *Each profile is featured here in gratitude for this financial support of the project.*

NASHVILLE ACADEMY OF MEDICINE

Past Presidents

Year	President		Year	President
1943	Henry L. Douglass, M.D.*		1976	Dan S. Sanders, Jr., M.D.
1944	Murray B. Davis, M.D.*		1977	James W. Hays, M.D.
1945	Beverly Douglas, M.D.*		1978	John L. Sawyers, M.D.
1946	George K. Carpenter, Sr., M.D.*		1979	Charles M. Hamilton, M.D.*
1947	John C. Burch, M.D.*		1980	B. F. Byrd, Jr., M.D.
1948	W. W. Wilkerson, Jr., M.D.*		1981	Robert W. Ikard, M.D.
1949	Daugh W. Smith, M.D.*		1982	Ronald E. Overfield, M.D.
1950	Cleo Miller, M.D.*		1983	Paul R. Stumb, M.D.
1951	R. H. Kampmeier, M.D.*		1984	John K. Wright, M.D.
1952	Hollis E. Johnson, M.D.*		1985	John B. Thomison, M.D.
1953	W.O. Terrill, Jr., M.D.*		1986	Kent Kyger, M.D.
1954	Charles C. Trabue, IV., M.D.*		1987	Sarah H. Sell, M.D.
1955	Robert N. Buchanan, Jr., M.D.		1988	James M. High, M.D.
1956	James C. Gardner, M.D.*		1989	Howard L. Salyer, M.D.
1957	William O. Vaughan, M.D.*		1990	T. Guv Pennington, M.D.
1958	William G. Kennon, M.D.		1991	R. Benton Adkins, Jr., M.D.
1959	Rollin S. Daniel, Jr., M.D.*		1992	Arthur G. Bond, M.D.*
1960	Thomas S. Weaver, M.D.*		1993	Reuben A. Bueno, M.D.
1961	Laurence A. Grossman, M.D.			
1962	Joseph M. Ivie, M.D.*			
1963	Walter Diveley, M.D.*			
1964	Addison B. Scoville, Jr., M.D.*			
1965	James N. Thomasson, M.D.*			
1966	William F. Meacham, M.D.			
1967	Greer Ricketson, M.D.			
1968	Luther A. Beazley, M.D.			
1969	Louis Rosenfeld, M.D.			
1970	Robert L. Chalfant, M.D.			
1971	Robert L. McCracken, M.D.			
1972	C. Gordon Peerman, M.D.			
1973	Frank C. Womack, Jr., M.D.			
1974	George W. Holcomb, Jr., M.D.			
1975	David R. Pickens, Jr., M.D.			

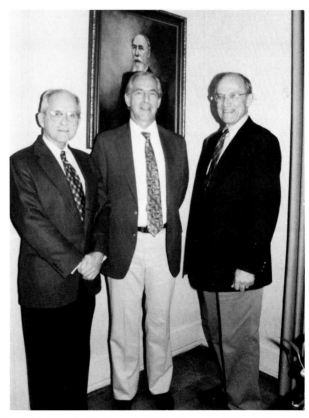

Left to right: Lonnie S. Burnett, M.D., President-Elect; David R. Yates, M.D., Chairman of the Board; John W. Lamb, M.D., President

1994	Barrett F. Rosen, M.D.
1995	Ann H. Price, M.D.
1996	John J. Warner, M.D.
1997	David R. Yates, M.D.
1998	John W. Lamb, M.D.

*deceased

Since its founding on March 5, 1821, the Academy has produced eight presidents of the American Medical Association:

1867	Paul F. Eve, M.D.
1875	William K. Bowling, M.D.
1890	William T. Briggs, M.D.
1913	John A. Witherspoon, M.D.
1925	W. D. Haggard, M.D.
1946	H. H. Shoulders, M.D.
1948	Olin West, M.D.
1978	Tom E. Nesbitt, Sr.

and forty three presidents of the Tennessee Medical Association:

James Roane, M.D.,	1830-32; 1832-34 (d.1833)
Felix Robertson, M.D.,	1834-36; 1836-38; 1838-40
Samuel Hogg, M.D.,	1840-42
A. H. Buchanan, M.D.,	1844-46; 1846-48

(Records for 1847, 1848, and 1849 have not been found)

Felix Robertson, M.D.,	1853-55
John P. Ford, M.D.,	1857-59
Charles K. Winston, M.D.	1859-61

(between 1863-66 no officers were elected due to war conditions)

Robert Martin, M.D.,	1866-67
J. D. Winston, M.D.,	1868-69
Joseph E. Manlove, M.D.,	1870-71
Paul F. Eve, M.D.,	1871-72
W. F. Glenn, M.D.,	1882-83
Thomas L. Maddin, M.D.	1885-86
W. T. Briggs, M.D.,	1886-87
Duncan Eve, M.D.,	1889-90
Giles C. Savage, M.D.,	1895-96
Deering J. Robert s, M.D.,	1901-02
Paul F. Eve, M.D.,	1904-05
A.B. Cooke, M.D.,	1907-08
John A. Witherspoon, M.D.,	1910-11
W. D. Haggard, M.D.,	1913-14
Charles N. Cowden, M.D.,	1916-17
H. M. Tigert, M.D.,	1922-23
W. C. Dixon, M.D.,	1925-26
Robert Cardwell, M.D.,	1931
J. O. Manier, M.D.,	1934
L. W. Edwards, M.D.,	1940
O. N. Bryan, M.D.,	1943
C.M. Hamilton, M.D.,	1946
Nat S. Shofner, M.D.,	1949
Daugh W. Smith, M.D.,	1952
Charles C. Trabue, M.D.,	1955
James C. Gardner, M.D.,	1958
William O. Vaughan, M.D.,	1961
Rudolph H. Kampmeier, M.D.,	1964
Tom E. Nesbitt, M.D.,	1970
O. Morse Kochtitzky, M.D.,	1973
C.Gordon Peerman, M.D.,	1976
James W. Hays, M.D.,	1979
George W. Holcomb, Jr., M.D.,	1982
John B. Thomison, M.D.,	1988
Howard L. Salyer, M.D.,	1991
R. Benton Adkins, Jr., M.D.,	1997

Georgina Abisellan, M.D.

Dr. Abisellan had originally wanted to be an attorney and to enter the diplomatic corps of her native Cuba. But her father was a physician and a dentist, and he hoped his only child would follow in his footsteps. He gently questioned her career choice, pointing out that no one in the family had ever been in politics, and steered her toward medicine.

She received her bachelor's degree from the Institute of Manzamillo Oriente at 17, then in 1960 graduated from Havana University's School of Medicine. Her residency was in ophthalmology, and she credits Professor Rodrigues Muro for kindling her interest in it. After two years private practice she and her family fled Castro's communist tyranny, abandoning all their possessions.

On reaching Nashville with her three small children, she had to find work. Because it would require years to validate her ophthalmology credential, she took a position at a local mental hospital. "While there I was incredibly fortunate to meet Drs. Nat Winston, Frank Luton, William Tragle, and, later, Drs. William Orr and Marc Hollender," she recalls. Dr.

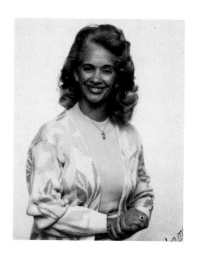

Abisellan subsequently completed a psychiatric residency at Vanderbilt. "I was blessed with supervisors such as Drs. Joseph Fishbein and Richard Stuart," she adds.

Today, Dr. Abisellan is in private practice and also serves as clinical director of the psychiatric unit at Summit Medical Center. In the community, she is active in the YMCA and Holy Rosary Academy.

Dr. Abisellan's eldest son, Raul, is also a physician. Middle child Georgina is a member of Dr. Abisellan's practice. Youngest daughter Maria, an aeronautical engineer, works on the Venture Star project that will be launched to the moon in 1999. The doctor's beloved grandchildren include Christopher, Lauren, and David.

Edward E. Anderson, M.D.

A saddlebag in Dr. Anderson's proud possession belonged to his grandfather, a physician in Forrest, Mississippi. There are four generations of the Anderson family in medicine, including Dr. Anderson's father and uncle, a brother, and a nephew.

During his training at Vanderbilt Medical School (1958-61) and postgraduate residencies and fellowships at the University of Virginia (1967-69), Dr. Anderson witnessed the evolution of cardiology into a subspecialty of internal medicine. "Invasive procedures separated the two," he recalls today.

In 1969 he became cardiologist in the cardiovascular laboratory at St. Thomas Hospital, the only hospital with a catheter laboratory. Two other doctors worked with him there. In two-and-one-half years, the lab saw a thousand cases. Now it sees 7,000 a year, and such facilities exist in many other local and regional institutions.

Dr. Anderson's colleagues in cardiology now number thirty eight. Dr. Anderson helped to set up coronary care units in surrounding towns, including Gallatin, Lewisburg,

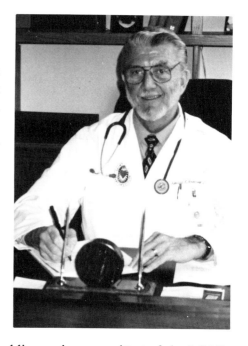

and Springfield. In those days, patient measurements from these sites came to him over the telephone, hooked to a tracing machine.

In addition to membership in local, state, and national medical societies, Dr. Anderson has served the profession as chairman of the public service committee of the Middle Tennessee Heart Association. In the years between medical school and residency, he saw service as a flight surgeon in the United States Navy, aboard the U.S.S. Saratoga, and with the First Marine Air Wing in Viet Nam.

PETER N. ARROWSMITH, M.D.
ARROWSMITH EYE INSTITUTE

Motivated in his career choice by a wish to help people, Peter Arrowsmith decided during his medical school years at the University of Miami that he wanted a surgical specialty. He interned at Vanderbilt University School of Medicine, completed his residency in ophthalmology there, going on to serve as chief resident.

Dr. Arrowsmith specializes in eye surgery, in the subspecialities of refractive, cataract, and implant surgery with a particular emphasis on corneal, refractive, and lens implant surgeries to correct nearsightedness, farsightedness, and astigmatism. He has done extensive work in the area of refractive surgeries, including coauthoring a textbook on refractive surgery, plus other publications. Dr. Arrowsmith is board certified through the American Board of Ophthalmology. He has served medical director at the Arrowsmith Eye Institute since 1977.

The Arrowsmith Eye Institute offers vision correction options for myopia and astigmatism. These procedures, known as Laser Assisted In-situ Keratomileusis (LASIK) and Photorefractive Keratectomy (PRK), utilize the Excimer laser located in the Institute's surgery center. In LASIK, the newer procedure, the surgeon uses a motor-powered blade called a microkeratome to partially detach a hair-width flap of the corneal membrane. After the flap is laid back, the laser remodels the corneal tissue underneath. The flap is then folded back into place, no stitches needed. The eye's membrane heals quickly, and vision is usually restored in a day.

Besides his busy practice, Dr. Arrowsmith is active in organized medicine. Among many such positions, he has served on the membership services committee and formerly as co-chairman of the nominating and membership committee of the National Academy of Eye Surgeons. He has held the post of medical director of the Eye Surgery Center of Middle Tennessee since 1984.

Dr. Arrowsmith's wife, Barbara, is an operatic singer, who has performed with the Nashville Symphony, the Nashville Opera, and other ensembles. Daughter Kelly recently graduated from the University of Findlay and trains high-performance horses. Son Kevin is following in his mother's footsteps, being a student of music theory and composition at Middle Tennessee State University.

Dr. Arrowsmith's associates at Arrowsmith Eye Institute include Norris L. Newton, M.D., and James S. Eubank, O.D.

Dr. Norris Newton is a board-certified ophthalmologist and medical graduate of the University of Oklahoma with specialty training at the Johns Hopkins Wilmer Eye Institute. He has served with U.S. Air Force Medical Corps of the U.S. Air Force and as chief of the ophthalmology research branch of the School of Aerospace Medicine. Dr. Newton is author of clinical, scientific, and research publications.

Dr. James Eubank, is the Institute's clinical coordinator. He specializes in general eye care with an emphasis on vision correction and treats glaucoma, infections, and injuries. He is a graduate of Southern College of Optometry in Memphis. Prior to entering private practice, he served in the U. S. Army Medical Service Corps, including time assigned to Fort Campbell. Dr. Eubank is a long-time officer in the Tennessee Academy of Optometry.

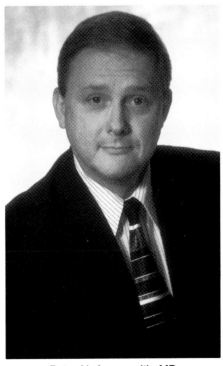

Peter N. Arrowsmith, MD

Associates in Gastroenterology

Established to assist patients with problems involving the digestive system, Associates in Gastroenterology comprises Dr. Whit James, Dr. Sue Lee, and Dr. Donald Lazas.

Dr. James' grandfather and father were physicians. He chose medicine because it blended science (his favorite school subject) and the art of communication. He received his medical degree from Wake Forest University. Dr. Willis Maddox, chairman of the department of medicine, influenced Dr. James to specialize in gastroenterology, and he completed a fellowship at Rush University. Dr. James is board-certified in both internal medicine and gastroenterology. He enjoys family activities, gardening, and swimming, and is active in the Nashville Academy of Medicine's Doctors in the Classroom series.

Dr. Lee is a native of Korea. She received her medical degree from Emory University in Atlanta, where she also completed a fellowship in gastroenterology. She numbers among her outstanding teachers Dr. Jonas Shulman ("an excellent clinician; intelligent; caring; a no-nonsense approach—and lots of common sense"). Before starting private practice, Dr. Lee taught at Emory University and Vanderbilt University. She is board-certified in internal medicine and gastroenterology. Dr. Lee's husband, Dr. R. Mickey Wheatley, is a cardiologist at St. Thomas. They have two children.

Dr. Lazas is a native of Washington, D.C., and received his medical degree at George Washington University. He counts Dr. Richard Snell, his anatomy professor, as his most memorable teacher. Pursuing a fellowship in gastroenterology at Walter Reed Army Medical Center, he met his mentors, including Drs. Roy Wong, Barry Marshall, and Willis Maddrey. Dr. Lazas is board certified in internal medicine and gastroenterology and a fellow of the American College of Physicians. He and his wife, Kathy, have five children.

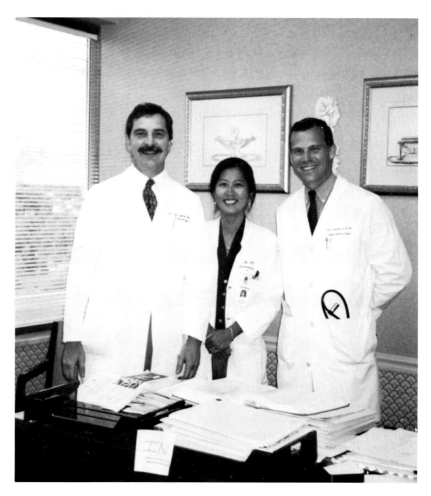

Left to right: Dr. Whit James, Dr. Sue Lee, and Dr. Donald Lazas

CHARLES BECK, M.D.

In Silsby, Texas, where he grew up, Charles Beck learned from his parents to revere study and learning. "I wanted a challenging field," he recalls, "one where I could also give myself in service to other people."

At the Baylor University's medical school, he recalls especially Dr. James K. Alexander, teacher of physical diagnosis, and Dr. Michael DeBakey, who told students, "There's an excuse for being ignorant, but none for not being thorough." Another teacher, Hebble Hoff, the head of the physiology department, made a lasting impression on the young medical student.

The newly-minted physician visited his wife's home, Nashville, and met Dr. W. J. Card in Madison. The joint practice that emerged was a confederation but it had all the advantages of a partnership. It eventually included Drs. George Hagan and James High. Half of Nashville's population lived east of the Cumberland River, but these were among the very few internists in the section.

This nucleus formed the basis of Madison Hospital's internal medicine department, which Dr. Beck helped set up.

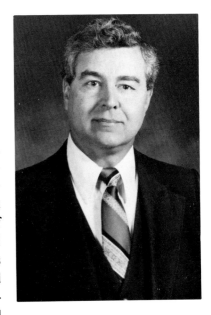

Dr. Beck is married to Angela Logan Beck, and they are the parents of Angela Sheryl Beck, Keith Bernard Beck, and Lisa Michelle Beck.

Dr. Beck has served on the Board of Trustees of Memorial Hospital for 17 years and is a member of the board of the Nashville Memorial Foundation. He belongs to Madison's Dellwood Baptist Church. In a recent interview he cited one of his favorite Bible verses, Ephesians 3:16, the prayer of the Apostle Paul: "That he would grant you, according to the riches of his glory, to be strengthened with might by his Spirit in the inner man."

H. VICTOR BRAREN, M.D.

Asked why he chose medicine as his life's work, Dr. Braren answered unhesitatingly, "I always wanted to help people." He received his M.D. degree from Tulane in 1968 and started his residency in urology at Charity Hospital in New Orleans. He remembers Dr. Jorgen U. Schlegel as a special influence there. He completed his residency in surgery and urology at Ohio State University Hospital and Columbus Children's Hospital before becoming, in 1973, the first pediatric urologist in Tennessee. He continues to limit his practice to this field today.

His research interests include fetal urology, pediatric urologic oncology, metabolic and growth problems secondary to urinary intestinal diversion, radioisotopic renal function, techniques for reconstruction of the external genitalia, and pediatric lower urinary tract urodynamics. He has received extensive grant support for work in certain of these areas and has published work in a wide range of medical journals and urology speciality publications.

Dr. Braren has faculty appointments at Vanderbilt and Meharry, has served on many hospital and university committees and in numerous societies and study groups. At the Nashville Academy of Medicine, he has chaired its legislative and governmental affairs committee.

From 1981-92, Dr. Braren served as advisor to Presidents Reagan and Bush for health-related appointments. He has

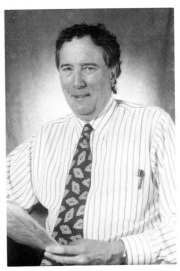

been a member of the national cancer advisory board of the National Cancer Institute. He has twice served as president of the Tennessee Urological Association and is a past president of the Nashville Surgical Society.

Dr. Braren and his wife, Judy, have three sons, Gary, Stephen, and David.

Baptist Hospital

Baptist Hospital, from its beginning, has been a Christian healing ministry committed to rendering the highest quality care in an exceptionally caring and compassionate atmosphere. On December 12, 1918, five men sought a charter of incorporation from the state to establish the Nashville Protestant Hospital. The urgent need for more hospital beds to serve Davidson County's growing population of almost 167,000 had become apparent with the devastating Spanish influenza epidemic. The $250,000 facility was an outgrowth of the Ministers Alliance of Nashville, which ruled that no physician would serve on the board of governors. Although the Protestant churches in the city shared decision making and management responsibilities, the hospital was interdenominational. The first patient was the newborn Margaret Anita Kilby Lewis, daughter of Gladys Kilby, and she arrived on March 20, 1919, two days before the official opening. The millionth patient was also a baby girl, Michelle Brinton, born in 1988.

The plot of ten-and-a-half wooded acres consisted of two adjoining city blocks, generally referred to as the Murphy Home Place, bounded by four streets: Church Street on the south, Twentieth Avenue on the east, Twenty-first Avenue on the west, and Patterson Street on the north. There were two buildings—one became the hospital and one became the dormitory for the school of nursing. Protestant Hospital began with 100 beds, and the construction of the East Building in 1924 increased capacity to 210 beds and 18 bassinets. Because of the Great Depression and generally weak financial condition, the hospital experienced no more growth.

Financial woes continued over the years until, threatened with bankruptcy, the hospital transferred ownership to the Tennessee Baptist Convention on April 11, 1948. The not-for-profit hospital changed its name to Mid-State Baptist Hospital. The Mid-State Baptist Hospital, Inc., School of Nursing was organized in June, 1948, following the dissolution of the original school at the time of the hospital's new ownership. During the 1940s and 1950s, the hospital added the south building, a new west building, the Ford Annex, an auditorium, and laundry and maintenance facilities.

The hospital progressed considerably in the 1960s and 1970s. A neonatal intensive care unit, called the Special Care Nursery, opened in 1961 and Nashville's first Coronary Care Unit, a first-step development of major cardiac surgery and diagnostic services, opened in 1964. That same year, the hospital became simply Baptist Hospital, Inc. Other significant developments were the additions of the Medical Intensive Care Unit and the Emergency Pavilion. By 1973, Baptist Hospital, Inc., with 600 beds had become the largest hospital in the mid-South. The purchase of St. Thomas Hospital's vacated Church Street property in 1975 enabled the establishment of the Progressive Care Center adding 108 rehabilitative beds. The center provided medical services for patients no longer needing acute care.

Baptist's leadership in health care and dedication to excellence became apparent in its 1980 founding membership in Voluntary Hospitals of America (VHA), an alliance of more than 1,200 not-for-profit health systems and hospitals to purchase supplies in a cost-effective way, and its 1984 creation of Health Net, an independent preferred provider organization. Medical milestones included implanting a nuclear-powered pacemaker in a patient in 1973, acquiring a total-body scanner using computerized axial technology (CAT) in 1976, and opening a lithotripter suite for the treatment of kidney stones in 1985. Baptist designed, equipped and staffed a specially designated surgery center for laser and laparoscopic surgery in 1990. The PET suite was constructed in 1996, housing a Positron Emission Tomography scanner for noninvasive cardiac imaging. Its goal is to diagnose disease early in order to lower risk and reverse heart disease.

Baptist has always sought to address all patient needs and has overseen many specialized care additions in the past decade. Centers of excellence include the Cancer Center, the Baptist Mind / Body medical institute (an affiliate program of Beth Israel Deaconess Medical Center and Harvard Medical School), the Neuroscience Center and occupational medicine and corporate health programs, the Mandrell Heart Center, the Orthopaedic Center, the Arthritis and Osteoporosis Care Center, the Diabetes Center, the Wound

Care Center, the Institute for Aesthetic and Reconstructive Surgery, the Rehabilitation Center, and Baptist Home Health Services.

The administrators, physicians, and board of trust at Baptist recognize that education, prevention and wellness play an essential role in health care. The Center for Health and Wellness provides educational classes for the community as well as health screenings, fitness testing, and other work-site wellness programs for businesses and organizations. On-site programs include group CPR classes, and classes on topics such as first aid, stress management, nutrition, and exercise; screenings for blood pressure and health risk appraisal; and flu shots and hepatitis B vaccinations. The Fitness Center and sports medicine program share similar goals of working to prevent future health problems among Middle Tennessee's amateur and professional athletes. The Women's Pavilion offers courses and care relating to parenting and childbirth.

Thanks to the hospital's visionary leaders, nearly $500 million in renovations have been added in the past eighteen years. Baptist Hospital is now licensed for 759 beds and covers 38 acres in its 50 Davidson County locations. The hospital's high-quality care resulted in a 1995 independent survey naming Baptist among the nation's top 100 Hospitals and in being recognized in 1996 and 1997 as a quality leader and preferred health care provider by the National Research Corporation. In 1997 Baptist offered hundreds of free public seminars and $26 million in uncompensated care.

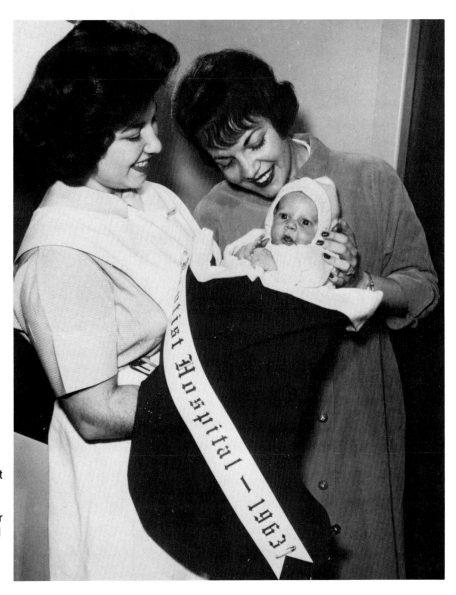

Mothers and fathers of babies born at Baptist Hospital during the week of Christmas bring home their "bundles of joy" in bright red Christmas stockings, like this mother and her newborn in 1963. The hospital has observed this tradition for more than 35 years.

HENRY B. BRACKIN, SR., M.D. AND HENRY B. BRACKIN, JR., M.D.

For 70 years this father-and-son team have practiced psychiatry with a specialty in adult psychiatry and management of major mood and thought disorders. Dr. Brackin, Sr., a fifth generation Sumner Countian, was born July 15, 1897, and graduated from the University of Tennessee School of Medicine in 1921. After interning at Nashville General Hospital, he trained in psychiatry at the King's Park State Hospital, Long Island, New York, and at the Dorothea Dix State Hospital, Raleigh, North Carolina. In 1928 he became assistant superintendent at Nashville's Central State Hospital.

A local pioneer in his field, Dr. Brackin was the first practitioner in Tennessee to use malaria fever therapy to treat central nervous system syphilis. While superintendent of the Davidson County Hospital between 1936 and 1944, he introduced in Tennessee the use of metrozole convulsive therapy for treating schizophrenia. He had never witnessed this procedure; only three other physicians in the nation had ever given it. Metrozole convulsive therapy preceded electro-convulsive therapy, and Dr. Brackin was also a pioneer in its use.

In 1944 Dr. Brackin entered private practice, admitting his patients at Madison Hospital. In association with Dr. Harry Witztum, he developed there the first insulin coma unit for schizophrenia in this area.

Dr. Henry B. Brackin, Jr. was born at the Dorothea Dix Hospital on November 3, 1924, and spent almost his entire childhood living on the grounds of state hospitals. After graduating from Vanderbilt's medical school, he trained in surgery before deciding to enter psychiatry. He did this specialty study at the U.S. Naval Hospital in Oakland,

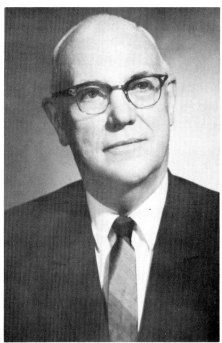

Henry B. Brackin, Sr.

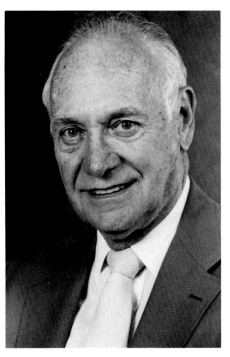

Henry B. Brackin, Jr.

California, and the hospital of the University of Pennsylvania. In 1954 he returned to Nashville, forming a private practice with his father. After his father's death in 1971, he was in partnership with Dr. William S. Sheridan, Jr., until 1992. Since then he has been a partner in Psychiatric Consultants.

In 1967 Dr. Brackin set up at Madison Hospital a clinical laboratory for measuring lithium and began the use of lithium in Middle Tennessee to treat manic depressive patients. In 1973 he and Dr. Charles B. Smith led the development of the Parthenon Pavilion at Centennial Medical Center. Dr. Brackin opened an insulin coma unit there, the last one in the United States to close as psychotropic medications came into general use. He served nine years as chief of the psychiatric staff; on the hospital's board of trustees for eighteen years; and as preceptor for electro-convulsive therapy. He has been an assistant clinical professor of psychiatry at Vanderbilt since 1964.

Father and son were founding members of the Tennessee Psychiatric Association in 1954, Dr. Brackin, Sr., serving as president in 1967. Between 1970 and 1974 lectures on schizophrenia were given in his honor at the University of Tennessee by outstanding researchers.

Dr. Brackin, Jr., has been president of the Tennessee Psychiatric Association, 1969; was a member of the executive committee of the assembly of the American Psychiatric Association, 1969-77; a member of that group's board of trustees, 1978-81; and president of the Southern Psychiatric Association, 1985. He has also served on several committees of the Tennessee Medical Association and the Nashville Academy of Medicine.

CARDIOVASCULAR SURGERY ASSOCIATES

Cardiovascular Surgery Associates is a professional corporation comprising board-certified thoracic surgeons who perform adult cardiac and thoracic surgery at St. Thomas Hospital.

Incorporated in 1974, this group was conceived in 1965 by Dr. William Stoney, who believed that open-heart surgery could be successfully performed in a private hospital in Nashville. Aided by Dr. George Burrus and Dr. William Alford, a heart-lung machine was purchased, laboratory experience acquired, and hospital approval obtained. In 1967 the first patient had his damaged mitral valve replaced with a Starr-Edwards prosthesis. From this initial success, the practice has grown to become one of the largest adult cardiothoracic surgical practices in the United States, with 14 surgeons performing a variety of procedures.

This group has done work in heart transplant, coronary artery bypass, pacemakers, tissue valves, transmyocardial laser revascularization, and minimally invasive operations on the heart, with and without the heart-lung machine. The first coronary artery by-pass and the first heart transplant in Tennessee were performed by this group. Other procedures routinely done are insertion of implantable defibrillators, repair of adult congenital heart problems, and repair or replacement of all heart valves, as well as the thoracic aorta. A thoracic oncology clinic under the direction of Dr. Jonathan Nesbitt brings together pulmonologists, medical oncologists, radiation oncologists, thoracic surgeons, and researchers to treat patients with lung and esophageal cancer. Clinical trials for newer therapies are adopted and utilized when approved by the Institutional Review Board of the hospital, and results are reported at regional and national meetings.

Throughout the years, the practice has emphasized refining members' surgical techniques, utilizing new technological breakthroughs, and the continual training of nurses and ancillary personnel involved with the care of patients.

Cardiovascular Surgery Associates works in a challenging and satisfying field of medicine and for more than 30 years has contributed to the progress of this speciality in Middle Tennessee.

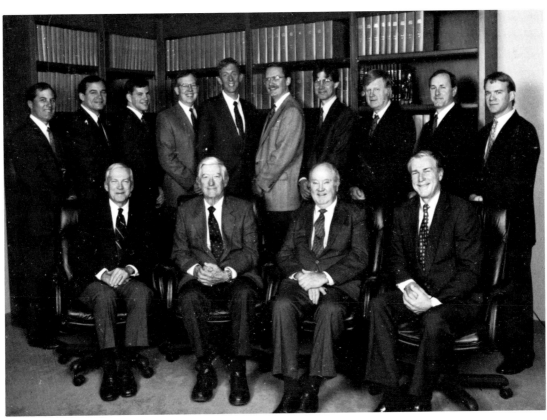

The physicians of Cardiovascular Surgery Associates

GERALD R. BURNS, M.D.

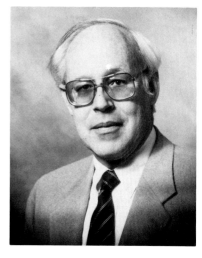

Dr. Burns' family has maintained its farm in Townsend for six generations, but coming of age in the Sputnik era the young man became interested in science and decided he preferred a people-oriented profession. His parents shared his vision and an uncle also influenced him. "He was an old-time doctor who made house calls and sometimes accepted chickens in payment. That kind of service mentality makes medicine a profession."

After doing all his undergraduate and medical school years at the University of Tennessee, graduating in 1966, Dr. Burns chose his specialty. He completed his surgical residency in 1972, then served two years in the U. S. Air Force.

Among the faculty at UT whom he remembers best is Dr. William Woods, professor of pharmacology. "As a subject, it's largely memory work, but Dr. Woods was a bright, shining light as a teacher," Dr. Burns recalls. Like all UT-trained surgeons, he also speaks with great respect for Dr. Louis Britt.

Dr. Burns has been in the practice of general surgery in Nashville since August, 1974. He was a trustee at Donelson Hospital from 1984-94 and chairman from 1990-94. In May, 1995, he began a three-year term on the board of the Summit Medical Center. He also serves as a trustee of the Donelson Primary Care Network, a part of the Columbia Healthcare Network.

Dr. Burns' wife, Sherry, manages his office and, being a nurse, assists him in surgery. Their children are Steven, an attorney in Washington, D.C.; Kenneth, attending graduate school at the University of Chicago; and Bonnie, a student at Belmont University.

WILLIAM GRAY DAVIS, M.D.

Dr. Davis looks back on the days when he worked alongside his grandfather, a Tennessee dairy farmer. "He had always wanted to become a doctor," Dr. Davis recalls, "and by the time I was 11 years old he had persuaded me in that direction."

As a youngster, he attended Catholic schools, and counts as his formative influences the nuns who "gave me love and attention, making me love school." He graduated from Howard High School in south Nashville, then won a bachelor's degree at Vanderbilt in 1961. He trained at the University of Tennessee medical school and interned at John Gaston Hospital in Memphis. He returned to Vanderbilt for his residency, "because Nashville was my home town and I wanted to continue my roots in this area."

Inclined to an interest in surgery, Dr. Davis selected a speciality in problems of the ear, nose, and throat. "It offered both medical and surgical exposure," he notes.

In organized medicine, Dr. Davis has been president of the Nashville Society of Otolaryngology and Opthalmology,

and chief of the department of Eye, Ear, Nose, and Throat at Memorial Hospital on three occasions. He served as president of the Nashville Memorial Hospital staff from 1993 to 1995. He is board-certified in otolaryngology, is a member of the American Academy of Otolaryngology and a Fellow of the American College of Surgeons.

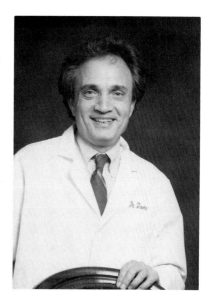

Dr. Davis' older son, Stan, practices law. His younger brother, Shane, works for the United States Postal Service. Dr. Davis and wife Glenna have a daughter, Parker.

G. WILLIAM DAVIS, M.D.

Whenever his uncle Dr. Robert Shands would invite young Bill Davis to observe surgery, the lad eagerly accepted. He was still an adolescent, but he often returned home smelling of ether.

Well before he finished high school, there in his hometown of Tupelo, Mississippi, he knew exactly what his calling was. In a recent interview, he recalled Martin Luther's observation that "a vocation is a sign of God's grace. I feel that way. As a very young man, I was focused on what I wanted to do, and I have kept that focus to this day."

Following three years of undergraduate study at Vanderbilt University, young Davis entered medical school at Emory, where he received the M.D. degree in 1957. He remembers with special regard a professor of physiology, Dr. Arthur Guyton, who told students, "Half of what I'm teaching you today is wrong. We just don't know which half."

Dr. Davis's internship and general surgical residency were done at Mid-State Baptist Hospital. Dr. Davis then returned to Vanderbilt for a three-year residency in orthopaedic surgery. There he studied under chief of surgery Dr. William Hillman and with noted Nashville physicians Drs. Ben Fowler and Eugene Regen.

In 1963 Dr. Davis set up his private practice near the campuses of Vanderbilt and Baptist Hospital. While carrying on an active practice, he would travel extensively as a lecturer for the next thirty-five years. He has visited some thirty countries to speak on aspects of spinal disease or injury, present demonstrations, or do surgery. He has also taught at the Vanderbilt University School of Medicine and served a guest teaching appointment in the radiology department of the University of California, San Francisco.

Dr. Davis has produced a film on the technique of surgical laserscope discectomy and published articles in the scientific literature of spinal surgery. He manages an occasional game of golf or tennis.

His office today is within a few blocks of his original location, and Dr. Davis retains the enthusiasm for medicine that he first gained in Dr. Shand's operating theater. "I love coming to work every morning!" he declares. "These spinal problems that people present never cease to fascinate me." He is currently engaged exclusively in the practice of lumbar spine surgery.

Dr. Davis's prime hospital affiliation is at Centennial Medical Center, and he enjoys courtesy staff privileges at St. Thomas and Park View. He holds board certification from the American Academy of Orthopaedic Surgery and the American Board of Orthopaedic Surgery. Active in organized medicine, he is an active member of the Nashville Academy of Medicine, the Tennessee Medical Association, the Nashville Surgical Society, the Tennessee Orthopaedic Society, among others.

ROBERT M. DIMICK, M.D.

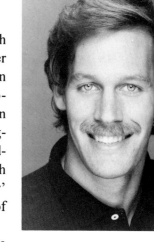

The son and nephew of physicians, Bob Dimick credits them with influencing him in the choice of medicine as a career. His father, Alan D. Dimick, practiced in their hometown of Birmingham. His great aunt Elizabeth Talley graduated from Tulane's medical school, becoming in the 1930s a pioneer woman physician in the South.

Dr. Dimick's mother encouraged his interests in sports, which ultimately led to his specialty in orthopaedic and spine surgery. "She had a good understanding of the balance between the sciences and the humanities," Dr. Dimick recalls. "She taught me that they complement each other."

Dr. Dimick was a scholarship varsity swimmer for the University of Alabama. The year he entered medical school, 1980, he also qualified for the swimming trials for the Olympics. His chances were thwarted when President Carter cancelled U.S. participation in the games.

An athletic injury led him to therapy with orthopaedic surgeons at the University of Alabama Hospitals. He later studied the science with Frank Owens, a lawyer as well as a physician and chief of orthopaedics at Lloyd Nolan Hospital in Birmingham. Dr. Dimick credits his mentor with "teaching me the 'why' as well as the 'how' of orthopaedics."

Since his orthopaedic residency, Dr. Dimick has held fellowships in knee surgery, sports medicine, and spinal surgery. Between 1992 and 1994, in private practice in Pensacola, he served as team physician at the University of West Florida. Since August of 1994 he has been in private practice in Nashville.

J. EMMETT DOZIER, JR., M.D.

Dr. Dozier comes from a family of physicians. His grandfather, Dr. William Bate Dozier, founded Nashville's Dozier Hospital.

He attended Vanderbilt from undergraduate years through medical school. During the latter, he became "captured," he says, by pediatric and child psychiatry. He recalls Dr. William Orr, the chairman of the department of psychiatry, as a mentor who encouraged his research interests and worked with him to publish. Dr. Dozier was inclined to enter private practice, but Dr. Hank Coppolillo, head of the division of child psychiatry, persuaded him to continue in academic medicine.

Holding various titles, between 1978 and 1986, Dr. Dozier directed Vanderbilt Medical Center's division of child and adolescent psychiatry and served as first medical director of the Child and Adolescent Psychiatric Hospital.

Today, in addition to maintaining an office in the community, he serves as clinical director of the child psychiatry unit at the hospital. He and some of his colleagues have been together for 20 years. Dr. Dozier counts as the great pleasures of his work the chance to help train the young doctors

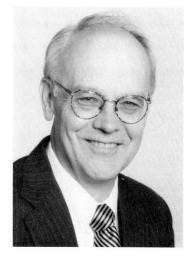

doing fellowships in child psychiatry and, of course, working with children and their families. In 1992 the child psychiatric residents established the J. Emmett Dozier Award, presented each year in recognition of dedication, compassion, service, and excellence in teaching.

Dr. Dozier has been president of the Tennessee Academy of Child Psychiatry, president of the Tennessee Society for Adolescent Psychiatry, and a fellow of the American Psychiatric Association.

Dr. Dozier is married to Louise Davis Dozier ("my childhood sweetheart"), and they are the parents of Louise and Chip. Dr. Dozier is a charter member of the Episcopal Church of the Resurrection in Williamson County.

Lloyd C. Elam, M.D.

Dr. Elam traces the roots of his vocation in psychiatry to Kretchner's *Personality and Physique*, which he read as an adolescent. Kretchner argued that the latter strongly influences the former. "I became fascinated by the question, 'What is the relation between the body and the mind?'" Dr. Elam recalls today. "I read and read, and by junior high school, I had decided on medicine, because I wanted to do research in this area."

He attended Roosevelt University in Chicago as an undergraduate and in 1957 received the M.D. degree from the University of Washington School of Medicine. He returned to the Midwest, to the University of Illinois at Chicago, to serve an internship. His developing research interests—including psychosomatic medicine and the state of mental health services in the nation's general hospitals—took him to the University of Chicago for residency training in psychiatry.

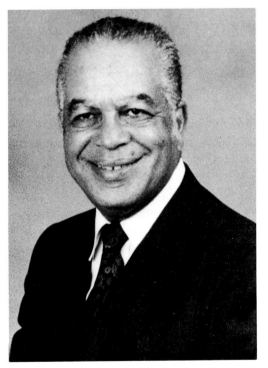

While doing his residency he taught a course in depression. At the time it was widely thought that manic-depressive illness was rare, except in Alabama and Tennessee. Researchers in those states—in Tennessee, Dr. Frank Luton—had conducted extensive epidemiological studies, which had not been done elsewhere.

"We know now," observes Dr. Elam, "that this illness exists all over the world. But when I had a chance to come to Tennessee, this 'fact' intrigued me." Dr. Matthew Walker, professor of surgery at Meharry, met Dr. Elam on a visit to Chicago and in 1961 the young physician became staff psychiatrist at George W. Hubbard Hospital. He subsequently established Meharry's department of psychiatry (behavioral studies having been formerly lodged in internal medicine). From 1963-68 he served as professor and chairman, and in 1966-68 took the post of interim dean of Meharry's school of medicine.

In September, 1967, Meharry's board of trustees elected him president of the College. In his inaugural address he announced plans for $30 million worth of new facilities, including a new Hubbard Hospital, computer center, allied health professions building, dental school, and a dozen more. Between then and 1976, Meharry's centenary, Dr. Elam oversaw the building of a virtually new campus. He resigned as president in 1981, served a year as Meharry's chancellor, then returned to the classroom.

Dr. Elam has been active in organized medicine and held membership, offices, and directorships of many civic, educational, and business enterprises, local and national. These last include serving on the boards of Fisk University and the Nashville Mental Health Association. He has been a member of the national advisory council to the National Institute of Mental Health and was appointed by President Lyndon B. Johnson to the national advisory committee to the Commission on Population and Planning. His has received honorary doctorates from Harvard University, St. Lawrence University, and Roosevelt University.

Dr. Elam's wife, Clara, is a retired pediatric nurse. Their older daughter, Gloria Elam, M.D., an obstetrician, is currently helping to establish a clinic for women in Uzbekistan. Her younger sister, Laurie Evans, Ph.D., works at the Center for Disease Control and teaches at Morehouse University.

KAREN B. DUFFY, M.D.

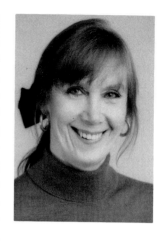

An interest in "figuring out how living things work" led Dr. Duffy to her vocation. Growing up in Chattanooga, she had a love for wildlife. About the time she entered the University of Chattanooga, her secondary school biology teacher, Betty Lackey, joined the faculty there. "She gave me the confidence to 'go for it' and was my most influential teacher," Dr. Duffy recalls.

At the University of Tennessee Graduate School of Medical Science, she studied immunology and microbiology. The isolated life of the laboratory wasn't for her, however. "I am gregarious, and I wanted to interact with people," she remembers. In 1970 she entered UT's College of Medicine.

Among her remembered teachers was Dr. Brusch, who taught her neuroanatomy ("a gentleman, very learned, very kind"), and the instructor who reassured her, when she fainted in anatomy, that one of the finest surgeons the institution had ever produced had done the same thing.

Following an internship at Memphis' Methodist Hospital, Dr. Duffy began practice as an emergency physician. After moving to Austin in 1978, she began working in one of the first walk-in clinics in the country. In 1982, having relocated to Nashville, she and three other doctors founded Nashville's Immediate Care Medical and Trauma Center, later Convenient Care. In 1983 she decided to pursue a solo practice and founded Madison Minor Medical Center, an outpatient medical center treating acute illness, injury, worker's compensation cases, and providing general practice. Madison Minor Medical Center is one of the very few independent clinics still in existence in the Nashville area.

"Minor emergency clinics have integrated well into the health care system," she observes. "At one time the emergency room was the source of primary care for many patients, but they might wait 12 hours for attention to a non-life-threatening problem."

Dr. Duffy and her husband, Ted Kromer, are active members of the Nashville Ballet, the Nashville Symphony, and Cheekwood. They have four children, Chris, Edward, Erin, and Jennifer.

GEORGE D. HAGAN, M.D. AND JOHN B. HAGAN, M.D.

Dr. George Hagan attributes his interest in medicine to having grown up in a home where doctors' families lived on either side; Dr. John Hagan shared a roof with his exemplar, his dad. "I was toting a doctor's bag and beginning to give injections to oranges by age three," the younger man says with a smile.

Dr. George's birthplace was Tompkinsville, Kentucky. He did undergraduate work at George Peabody College. Applying to the University of Tennessee medical units, he was told that the only remaining openings were in dentistry or pharmacy. "No, I want to be a physician," he insisted. A week later, the school called to offer him a place in the Class of '53.

During an internship at St. Thomas, Dr. George studied with Dr. William R. Cate, an internist who had one of the early electriocardiagram machines. Dr. Cate's associate was Dr. Addison Scoville.

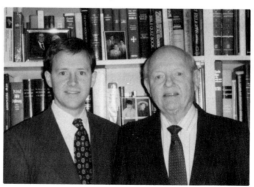

Drs. John B. and George B. Hagan

Among his mentors, Dr. George also names Dr. Thomas Frist, Sr. After military service Dr. Hagan opened a private practice in Madison, joining Dr. William J. Card in August, 1959.

His partner is his protege, Dr. John. He was an undergraduate at Baylor, won his medical degree at the University of Tennessee, and did postgraduate training at the Mayo Clinic. This last included fellowships in allergy / immunology and critical care medicine. One of his best-remembered teachers there was Dr. Stewart Nunn, a cardiologist and classmate of Dr. George.

Dr. George Hagan is married to Mary Fandrich. Besides Dr. John, their children are Mary Jane Hagan Evans and Joseph Fandrich Hagan. Dr. John's wife is Julianne Raines Hagan, and their children are Bethany Grace Hagan and Christian Raines Hagan.

Fred Goldner, M.D.

"The ability to help people integrated into what you do every day is a blessing," Dr. Goldner says about his work. "The course of my professional career has been a fortunate and inspiring journey."

Medical school at Vanderbilt University followed by internships at Piedmont Hospital in Atlanta and Boston City Hospital and residencies in internal medicine at Peter Bent Brigham (Brigham Women's Hospital) in Boston and Vanderbilt Medical Center laid the foundation for a lifetime of learning.

On assignment from Brigham Hospital for the U. S. Army, Dr. Goldner served with the surgical research unit at Fort Sam Houston in San Antonio. There he started armed services' first artificial kidney unit. Later Dr. Goldner set up such a unit in Nashville. For a time he served as the medical consultant for the kidney transplant program at Nashville Veteran's Administration Hospital.

Intensive experience with disease outcomes that did not present immediately have led him to name his practice The Center for Difficult Diagnosis, with specialties in hypertension, internal medicine, and prevention cardiology. Dr. Goldner declares that he gets "tremendous excitement" out of differential diagnosis.

At Vanderbilt University Medical Center, Dr. Rudolph Kampmeier transmitted to students the fine points of physical diagnosis. Dr. Goldner was also influenced by the teaching of Maimionides, who admonished doctors to recognize what may be comprehended even though absent or hidden: "To see what cannot be seen, for the delicate and indefinite indices must be given thoughtful deliberations in order to preserve lives and health."

While studying the work his patients could hope to do after a heart attack or surgery, Dr. Goldner observed, "Many of them would not have had heart disease in the first place if their blood pressure had been controlled." He continued, "I have always been interested in risk factors—exercise, lipids, lifestyle, and attitudes. If we can teach awareness, prevention, and responsibility for what individuals put into their mouths— food, drugs, cigarettes—we will see a lot less of these people later."

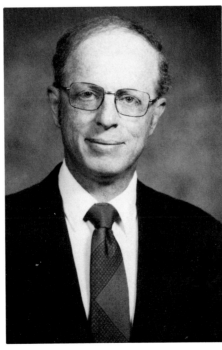

He has published laboratory and clinical studies on progressive systemic sclerosis (scleroderma), hypernatremia, azotemia and acidosis after cerebral injury, the artificial kidney, and a review of the transasscination reaction and its relationship to acute myocardial infarction.

Dr. Goldner has been an associate professor of clinical medicine at Vanderbilt University Medical Center and served as assistant clinical professor at Meharry Medical College. He is a Fellow of the American College of Physicians and the American College of Cardiology. He helped found the American Society of Hypertension and belongs to the American Society of Nephrology.

Dr. Goldner's community health activities are spread among the American Red Cross, the Cumberland Science Museum, the National Kidney Foundation, and the American Cancer Society. He is a past president of the Tennessee Diabetes Society, the Nashville Cardiovascular Society, and the Upper Cumberland Medical Society. He has served as vice president of the Middle Tennessee Heart Association.

Keeping Dr. Goldner's life and career within reason are his wife, Martha, and four children. In his life, family and practice have been central, enriched by personal passions of reading, jogging, cartooning, golf tee practice, following the Red Sox, and being with friends.

C. K. Hiranya Gowda, M.D.

Dr. Gowda was born in 1934 to Sri Krishne and Smit Krisnamma Gowda in Chamaraddahally, Mulbagel Taluk, Karnataka State, India. According to his father, who passed away in April 1995 at age 101, Chamaraddahally had been a village of about 134 people in 1934.

The youngster's parents taught him and five siblings their alphabets in Kannada and English. By age eight the children were walking six miles round trip to school. "It surprises me," Dr. Gowda recalls, "that we survived the cobras, bears, and occasional wild elephants that crossed our path through what was essentially a forest." Disease was another bane of childhood, Dr. Gowda observed. "I was lucky enough to escape the horrors of cholera, plague, smallpox, diphtheria, typhoid, and malaria, though some of my classmates departed to Heaven."

Finishing college, Hiranya Gowda entered the Mysore Medical College and completed his MBBS degree in 1960. He recalls the great influence of his anatomy professor, Dr. R. Y. Appajee. He completed an internship at Victoria Hospital in Bangalore, then returned to Mysore Medical College to teach pharmacology under the direction of Professor Dr. Ragunatha Rao.

In the fall of 1962 Dr. Gowda accepted a lectureship at the Bangalore Medical College, under the supervision of another mentor, Dr. H. Hiranniah. In the course of that work he decided to become an ear, nose, and throat surgeon. Between 1963 and 1969 he completed specialized training in St. Louis, Missouri, studying with Drs. Joseph Ogura and Joseph West. In 1970 Dr. Gowda came to Meharry Medical College as an assistant professor. He is now associate professor and division chief in otolaryngology. He holds the post of

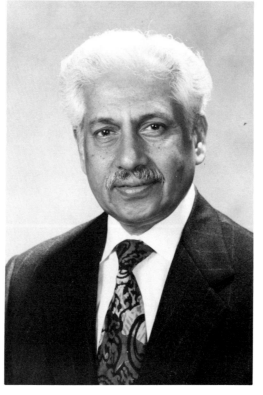

chief of otolaryngology and head and neck surgery at Nashville Metropolitan General Hospital. He is also clinical associate professor in the department of otolaryngology and head and neck surgery at Vanderbilt.

In addition to his professional practice, Dr. Gowda has a great range of business, religious and social-philanthropic interests. He has served as president of Incacomp Computer Center of Brentwood and of Nashville Hospitality Concepts. He co-founded the Hindu Cultural Center of Tennessee and served as chairman of the building committee of Sri Ganesha Temple. Since 1994 he has been chairman of the latter. Other community endeavors include service as president of the India Associations in both St. Louis (1966-67) and Nashville (1971-72).

Dr. Gowda contributes to community life in his home town as well as his adopted city. He is particularly interested in educational work, and has provided funding for two classrooms to Kambodi High School, Kolar Taluk. He contributes cash prizes for the top three students having the highest grades at twenty three high schools. Since the founding of these prizes, teachers report that grades have improved markedly.

He is also involved with an important preventive medicine project in his native village of Chamaraddahally, where in 1985 he completed the water supply system. It includes a bore well, a half-mile of piping, and a storage tank. Since the installation of the water supply system, there have been almost no gastroenteritis cases there.

Dr. Gowda married Saraswathi Devi in 1961, and they have two children: Manohar Sai Gowda, M.D., and Kalpana Kumari Gowda, Ph.D.

Herschel Graves, M.D.
Robert Sadler, M.D.

A native of Booneville, Mississippi, Dr. Bob Sadler traces his interest in medicine to the influence of Dr. William H. Anderson, whom he regarded as a hero and role model. Dr. Anderson owned and published *The Mississippi Doctor* and served as president of the state medical society. On young Sadler's graduation from high school, the doctor gave him a copy of Rudolph Matas's *The Soul of the Surgeon*, and Dr. Sadler recently passed it on to Dr. Anderson's grandson, himself a new physician.

Dr. Sadler did his undergraduate study at Union University in Jackson, Tennessee, and Carson Newman College, in Jefferson City. From his medical school years at Vanderbilt, 1944-47, Dr. Sadler feels a special debt toward surgeon Barney Brooks, pathologist James Dawson, and bacteriologist John Buddingham. "They were hard on students, but they stimulated us to have thoughts of our own," Dr. Sadler recalls. Upon his graduation, Dr. Sadler became a chest resident at Vanderbilt, the first one there.

Dr. Sadler served in the U.S. Navy from 1949-52 has been active in various committees of the Nashville Academy of Medicine. He played an active role in the Tennessee Political Action Committee during the national debate over Medicare, 1964-65. He is assistant clinical professor of surgery at Vanderbilt and the University School of Medicine. He is board-certified in both surgery and thoracic surgery. Among his several hospital appointments have been a year as chief of surgery at Parkview Hospital and a decade as chief of surgery at Westside Hospital.

Dr. Sadler is a deacon at Christ Presbyterian Church. He is married to Ellen Russell Sadler, and their children are Jane Greenway, Fred Russell Harwell, James Harwell, Sam Harwell, IV, Sue Rinehardt, and Robert Sadler, Jr.

Dr. Herschel Graves says that he and Dr. Sadler have been "blessed to witness an explosion of scientific knowledge and unparalleled social progress and economic prosperity" in the past 50 years. He names antibiotics, antihistamines, cortisone, and hypertension medications. In his specialty field, he cites gastrointestinal endoscopy, advances in anesthetic agents, open-heart surgery, total joint replacement, laparoscopic surgery, stapling devices, and CAT and MRI scanning. In his early years, Nashville hospital patients were served mainly in semi-private rooms or wards, as opposed to all private rooms today. Other institutional changes that he has witnessed include the establishment of post-operative recovery units, intensive care and coronary care units, and the building of first-class emergency pavilions. In the social and political arenas, Dr. Graves has seen the spread of private insurance and the enactment of Medicare and Medicaid. "We are indebted to the faculty of the Vanderbilt School of Medicine who taught us medicine, surgery, and a work ethic," writes Dr. Graves. "We are equally indebted to our forebears and peers in town who welcomed and worked with us."

"With all of the good came the bad—advertising and marketing," Dr. Graves adds. "Still, professional ethics have remained high, and the town-and-gown relationship has continued to be good."

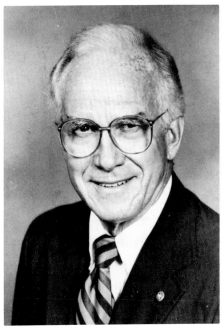

Dr. Hershel Graves

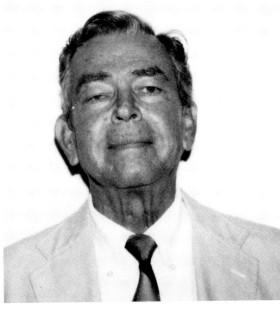

Dr. Robert Sadler

MARCUS C. HOUSTON, M.D.

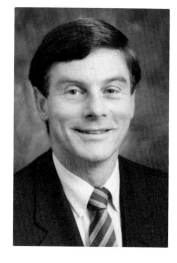

Mark Houston knew he wanted to be a doctor from the age of six. No family members had preceded him into medicine, nor was there a role model until he began to play school sports in his native Jackson. He and his teammates received Dr. Baker Hubbard's attention for sprained ankles or bruised elbows.

After an undergraduate career at Rhodes College, he entered Vanderbilt Medical School, where he met the two men he regards as mentors, Drs. Grant Liddle and Tom Brittingham. Although he urged young Dr. Houston to intern at Vanderbilt, Dr. Liddle assisted him in winning a place in his preferred program, the University of California Hospitals at San Francisco. Dr. Liddle recruited Dr. Houston to return to Vanderbilt as the Hugh J. Morgan Chief Resident for 1977-78. The third- and fourth-year medical students chose him as their best teacher, and he was presented the J. William Hillman Award for Excellence in Teaching.

Dr. Houston has held academic appointments at Vanderbilt since then. He is also director of the Hypertension Institute, St. Thomas Medical Group, St. Thomas Hospital.

Dr. Houston has written or co-authored books and monographs on hypertension and related diseases. He serves as an editorial consultant for various journals, including the *American Heart Journal*, the *American Journal of Medicine*, the *New England Journal of Medicine*, and others. Dr. Houston was elected a Fellow of the American College of Physicians in 1984.

He and his wife, Laurie (who serves as his nurse) have four children, Helen Ruth, Bo, John, and Kelly.

JOHN W. LAMB, M.D.

When he considered where he might practice, Dr. John W. Lamb chose Nashville because he had observed the quality of care available in almost any medical or surgical subspecialty. "If I couldn't find how to reach my objective with any patient," he recalls, "I could always find someone here who could help.

Born in North Carolina, John Lamb became captivated by science and medicine through an eighth-grade science class and books on the history of medicine and science, such as the popular treatises of Isaac Asimov. He did his undergraduate and medical school education at the University of Chicago, where he was exposed to the stories of great discoveries in orthopaedics by Drs. C. Howard Hatcher and Dallas B. Phemister. He particularly enjoyed the orthopaedic conferences, and during the last two years of medical school decided that would be the area where he most wanted to spend the rest of his life. He interned at Kings' County Hospital, in Brooklyn, New York, and served as a battalion surgeon with the 82nd Airborne Division, spending a year in the Dominican Republic.

Dr. Lamb's residency training was at the Albany Medical Center in New York. During the final year he had fellowships in Atlanta and in Nashville. His two most memorable teachers were Dr. Crawford J. Campbell, who encouraged him in learning the basic science of orthopaedics, and Dr. Benjamin Fowler, who encouraged him to use his ingenuity to make the solution fit the problem.

Dr. Lamb and his wife, Linda, have three children: John, in law school at the University of Chicago; Helena, working in the music business in Memphis; and Betsy, beginning college as a music major at the University of Michigan.

In 1998, Dr. Lamb became president of the Nashville Academy of Medicine. Of *Nashville Medicine: A History*, he says, "It attempts to delineate some of the contributions that this city has made to medicine in the entire country over many years. We can all be proud of the history of medicine in Nashville, and we should consider it a privilege to be a part of that distinguished tradition."

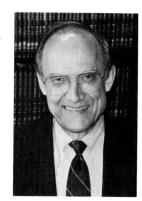

RALPH J. LANEVE, M.D.

Poet and pediatrician William Carlos Williams spoke of the *tactus eruditus*, the learned touch. Can fingers and hands inclined to an endeavor such as playing the guitar or laying a brick wall turn to a surgeon's intricate work?

Through high school in Pittsburgh and during college at the University of Pittsburgh, Ralph J. LaNeve set his sights on a career in music. Although his father was a pediatrician in private practice, he never considered medicine for himself.

Still, he had warm memories of accompanying his father on Sunday rounds at Children's Hospital, then going with the family to Forbes Field and a Pirates game. The young man's interest in music waned, and he took a degree *magna cum laude* in chemistry and won admission to Philadelphia's Jefferson Medical College. His stipend from the U.S. Army's Scholarship Program paid his way.

"Besides guitar, I'd done construction work through college. I framed houses, applied siding, installed new roofs. Once I decided on medicine, I knew absolutely that I wanted to do general surgery."

Dr. LaNeve did his internship and residency at the Letterman Army Medical Institute in San Francisco and was present there when the Loma Prieta earthquake struck in October, 1989. The base received the first casualties from the Marina district and the San Francisco Bay bridge collapse. "It was my first experience of trauma surgery," he recalls.

After five years at Letterman, Dr. LaNeve was assigned to the Irwin Army Community Hospital at Fort Riley, Kansas—in time for the Persian Gulf War. He traveled to the Mideast with civilian units from Texas and Oklahoma and took up his post as staff surgeon with the 44th Evacuation Hospital at King Kahlid Military City, Saudi Arabia. There he helped set up the sophisticated field hospitals that received the casualties from Operation Desert Storm.

During that assignment he heard a lot of contemporary, popular country music. It revived his interest in his old calling, and when he returned to the United States, he started playing instruments again. As he and his wife thought about a place to settle, they heard good things about Nashville, and he spoke with officials at the Donelson Hospital, then under construction, and accepted their offer of a position as house surgeon. He is currently in the private practice of general surgery, is a fellow of the American College of Surgeons, and a diplomate of the American Board of Surgery. He belongs to the Association of Military Surgeons and several medical societies including the Nashville Academy of Medicine.

Dr. LaNeve maintains his enthusiasm for music. His collection of classic guitars includes a '59 Les Paul and a '53 Telecaster. Son David is taking up base guitar and also plays baseball for the Brentwood Civitan team, where his father is an assistant coach.

Dr. LaNeve and his wife, Carol Rahme LaNeve, have two other children, Brenna and Matthew. Brenna is looking forward to joining her older brother on the ball team. The LaNeve family now makes its home in Brentwood.

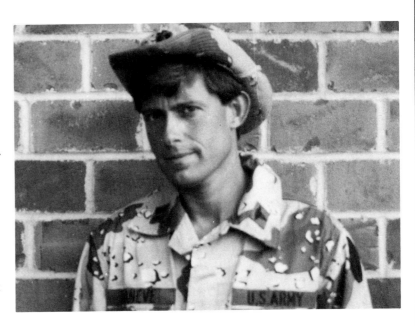

THE LIPSCOMB CLINIC

Dr. A. Brant Lipscomb, the founder of the Lipscomb Clinic, attended Vanderbilt University and served as team physician for Vanderbilt athletics for more than 40 years. In the 1950s he joined the Edwards-Eve Clinic in Nashville, across the street from St. Thomas Hospital.

The Lipscomb Clinic was founded in 1974 when Dr. Lipscomb, Sr., left the Edwards-Eve Clinic and joined with Dr. Robert K. Johnston and Dr. E. Dewey Thomas to start the Orthopaedic and Sports Medicine Surgery Practice, located in the St. Thomas Office Building.

Subsequently, Dr. Robert B. Snyder, Dr. Allen F. Anderson, Dr. William A. Shell, Jr., and Dr. A. Brant Lipscomb, Jr., joined the group. In 1990 the group relocated to the new St. Thomas Medical Plaza and changed its name to The Lipscomb Clinic in honor of Dr. Lipscomb, Sr.

Since that time Dr. Robert E. Clendidin, III, Dr. J. Keith Nichols, Dr. Michael J. Pagnani, Dr. David M. Schmidt, Dr. Edward S. Mackey, and Dr. Philip A. G. Karpos have joined the practice.

The Lipscomb Clinic is one of the most respected centers for sports medicine and orthopaedic surgery in the region. The spectrum of practice now includes sports medicine, hand surgery, spinal surgery, total joint replacement surgery, physical medicine and rehabilitation, and foot and ankle injuries, in addition to general orthopaedic care.

Today, Lipscomb Clinic has grown to eleven physicians: Allen F. Anderson, M.D.; Robert E. Clendidin, III, M.D.; Robert K. Johnson, M. D.; Philip A. G. Karpos, M.D.; Edward S. Mackey, M.D.; J. Keith Nichols, M.D.; Michael J. Pagnani, M.D.; Gregory W. Rennirt, M.D.; David M. Schmidt, M.D.; William A. Shell, M.D.; and Robert B. Snyder, M.D. In addition to the office at St. Thomas, The Lipscomb Clinic has had a second office on the Centennial Medical Center campus since 1997.

The Lipscomb Clinic is active in the medical research arena through the work of the Lipscomb Foundation for Research and Education, Inc., a nonprofit, tax-exempt organization created by Dr. Allen Anderson. The goals of the foundation are to facilitate scientific research and to provide a forum for the dissemination of knowledge acquired by research and to educate athletes, coaches, and physicians regarding the prevention and treatment of sports-related injuries.

In October, 1996, The Lipscomb Clinic joined with Tennessee Orthopaedic Associated to form Tennessee Orthopaedic Alliance. At the same time the new group became a founding practice in OrthoLink Physicians Corporation. OrthoLink in a physician-crafted, physician-directed management company that provides affiliated physicians the resources and infrastructure necessary to compete in the evolving healthcare marketplace.

MIDDLE TENNESSEE NEUROSURGERY

Neurological surgery is the discipline of medicine and that specialty of surgery that provides the operative and non-operative management of disorders of the central, peripheral, and autonomic nervous systems.

A single-specialty, professional service corporation, Middle Tennessee Neurosurgery provides services in the areas of neurosurgery. The practice comprises Drs. Arthur R. Cushman, Ronald T. Zellem, and Philip Rosenthal.

Dr. Cushman graduated from LaSierra University in Riverside, California, and Loma Linda University School of Medicine. He completed an internship in 1970 at the Los Angeles County University of Southern California Medical Center, returning to Loma Linda for residency training.

Dr. Cushman founded Middle Tennessee Neurosurgery, P.C., in 1975, then calling the practice Madison Neurological Services. In years past he has been chairman of the departments of neurosurgery and orthopedics at Nashville Memorial Hospital and Donelson Hospital. He is currently serving as president of the Tennessee Neurosurgical Association. He is a Diplomate of the American Board of Neurological Surgery. Dr. Cushman is married and has two children. His hobbies include collecting prehistoric American Indian artifacts and restoring passenger train cars and riding in them. In 1997-98 Dr. Cushman served as president of the Tennessee Neurosurgical Association.

In 1990 Dr. Cushman was joined by Dr. Zellem. A graduate of Emory University's medical school, he completed intern and residency training at Temple University in Philadelphia in 1976.

A Diplomate of the American Board of Neurological Surgery, Dr. Zellem has performed research in experimental peripheral nerve repair and in 1995 began performing modern pallidotomies for the surgical treatment of Parkinson's disease. He and his wife, Suzanne, have two children, Robert Thomas and Jennifer Suzanne. He enjoys guitar, model railroading, water sports and Civil War history. His interest in the last led him to serve as contributing editor of a reprinting of *The Medical and Surgical History of the Civil War* (Broadfoot Publishing, 1990-91).

In 1992 the corporation changed its name to Middle Tennessee Neurosurgery to accurately reflect the geographic area served. Two years later Drs. Cushman and Zellem acquired the services of Dr. Philip Rosenthal. He is a graduate of the Cornell University Medical College and completed his residency at the State University of New York. He also received fellowship training in spinal microsurgery. Like his colleagues, Dr. Rosenthal is a Diplomate of the American Board of Neurological Surgery. Dr. Rosenthal has done research on brain physiology and postoperative brain monitors. He and his wife have three children. Dr. Rosenthal enjoys classical music and is a licensed pilot.

The physicians of Middle Tennessee Neurosurgery have hospital privileges at Baptist Hospital, Summit Medical Center, Hendersonville Hospital, Nashville Memorial Hospital, Sumner County Regional Medical Center, and Tennessee Christian Medical Center.

Managing the overall operation of the practice is Mr. Christopher S. Davenport. He holds a bachelor in business administration degree from Belmont University and is a Certified Financial Planner and an Accredited Tax Preparer. In addition to the physicians and Mr. Davenport, Middle Tennessee Neurosurgery employs thirteen people in the areas of operations, administration, and nursing.

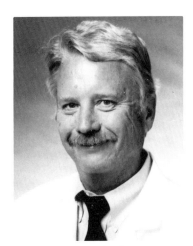

Dr. Arthur Cushman

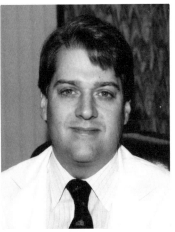

Dr. Ronald Zellem

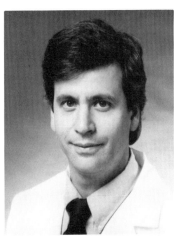

Dr. Philip Rosenthal

Metropolitan General Hospital

Once hailed by a local newspaper as a "magnificent city building" when it opened in 1890, as City Hospital, the now-named Metropolitan Nashville General Hospital proudly stands and actively administers quality health care for Nashville and surrounding communities. Concern for the welfare of the desperately ill or those unable to care for themselves motivated the community to establish a health care facility.

Even as early as 1823 Nashvillians advocated the building of a public hospital. Under the direction of Nashville's most prominent citizens, Boyd McNairy, Felix Roberton, James Overton, and James Roane, the State Legislature approved a lottery to raise money to build a new hospital. Despite their genuine cause and hard work, the lottery effort was deemed unsuccessful as insufficient funds were raised. Sixty-seven years passed before the city hospital was built when in 1879 the Nashville City Council finally authorized its construction. The site selected was the same place where in 1825, Marquis deLafayette landed and was greeted by Andrew Jackson.

Viewed as an elegant red brick building with towers, stone trim and arched windows sitting high on the bluffs of the Cumberland River, with "light airy rooms and lofty ceilings," the hospital opened on April 23, 1890 at a complete cost of $30,000. Dr. Charles Brower, a graduate of the University of Nashville, first supervised the 60-bed, four-ward hospital whose patients in that day and age were separated by gender and race. A small brick building housed the horse-drawn ambulances. To provide on-site training a school of nursing, then second in the nation, was added the same year and was under the direction of superintendent Charlotte E. Perkins. This was the first training school for nurses located between the Ohio River and New Orleans. The school closed in 1970.

In the late 1890s, City Hospital was staffed by Dr. Brower and seven nurses, five of which worked the 7:00 a.m. to 7:00 p.m. shift and two worked from 6:00 p.m. to 8:00 a.m. for $3.00 per day. Since there were no operating room nurses, the nurse in charge of a surgical patient would accompany the doctor during surgery.

The early 20th century brought much progress and development for City Hospital. In 1909, for example, sterilizers became part of routine hospital equipment and a new pediatric ward was created in 1914. In 1915, a new private wing was added; here student nurses participated in authentic hands-on private duty nursing training. The hospital's name was changed in 1923 to Nashville General Hospital.

Another wing was added in 1932 increasing the bed capacity to a total of 260. Until 1921 Dr. Brower treated all patients, and students and faculty from medical schools used the wards for teaching and learning. Then a new charter was written and a new hospital board appointed who invited leading specialists from Vanderbilt University and the community to help staff the hospital.

The hospital suffered from some erosion during World War II. Extensive remodeling occurred and modern equipment purchased when the city assumed operating the hospital and developed it into one of the finest in the area. In 1957 the hospital opened the first Well Baby Clinic in Nashville and started the School of Radiologic Technology. In 1970, Metro Nashville General Hospital performed a live-donor kidney transplant, the first done in Nashville. In 1976, the Maternal and Infant Care Program, a comprehensive health care program providing a wide range of services for mothers, fathers and their infants from prenatal stages until the infant reaches his second birthday was established. Also, in 1976, the Nuclear Medicine Clinic and a separate Metropolitan Employee Injured on Duty Clinic were built.

During the past two decades the hospital has expanded to meet the diverse needs of a growing city including: remodeling of Intensive Care Unit (1981); installation of the CAT SCAN (1982); the initiation of shared affiliation between Vanderbilt University Medical Center and Meharry Medical College (1985); opening of the Labor/Delivery/Postpartum rooms (1987); and the modernization of Outpatient Surgery Unit (1987).

To aid in strengthening the teaching bond and proximity to a medical college whose history and contributions reflect General Hospital's dedication to the citizens of Nashville, Metropolitan Nashville General Hospital relocated to Meharry Medical College campus in January, 1998. Since 1993 General has served as the clinical hospital for Meharry and has been staffed by Meharry physicians.

A three-year total renovation of the former George W. Hubbard Hospital began in 1994, and the new General Hospital has more than 350,000 square feet in its modernized facility, compared to some 150,000 at the Hermitage Avenue site.

Through the conversion of the former Emergency Room into a Primary Care Center serving a diversity of patient needs, the "grand lady" maintains a presence on Hermitage Avenue. Her mission still parallels her pioneer health care specialists' need to provide health care alongside community service. Today in accordance with the Charter of Metropolitan Government, the board of hospitals and the entire medical and hospital staff remain steadfast with their original mission:

> "To provide quality health care services to the Nashville/Davidson County Community, particularly the under-served, and also provide educational opportunities for the medical and allied health professions in a compassionate, ethical, and financially responsible manner."

The pioneering compassionate patient care exits today. During its centennial celebration, the Nashville community united to commemorate and honor the lives of their past caretakers who once walked the halls of the magnificent City Hospital. As Nashville approaches the 21st century, Nashville Metropolitan General Hospital, as a publicly-owned acute/primary healthcare system, provides acute tertiary care to patients of Bordeaux Hospital, Metro prisoners and detainees, Metro employees injured on duty, and the growing population of the Metropolitan Nashville and Davidson County area. With a commitment to the continuous improvement and excellence of all that they do, the staff of the Metropolitan General Hospital pledges to provide high quality, compassionate care and quality of life of all patients served. The vision and dedication of those who first created the hospital is still applauded over a century later.

MID-STATE ONCOLOGY AND HEMATOLOGY

Oncology is the science of caring for people with cancer and the planning of treatment options with them. Hematology is the science of the diagnosis and management of diseases of the blood.

Cancer is frightening to those whom it strikes, and the physicians and employees at Mid-State Oncology and Hematology try to make it less so. They seek to help the patient achieve physical and emotional healing, making possible a return to work, family, friends, and society. If a return to health is not possible, they assist the patient to find acceptance, and to ease suffering.

Mid-State Oncology and Hematology employs three physicians:

Michael J. Magee is a Donelson native. He received his B. S. degree from Auburn University and, in 1977, the M.D. degree from the University of Tennessee.

His medical oncology training was at Memorial Sloan-Kettering and his hematology training was at Vanderbilt. He is board certified in internal medicine, medical oncology, and hematology. He is also a Fellow in the American College of Physicians. He was recognized as teaching Attending for the Year at the University of Tennessee at Baptist Hospital internal medicine residency in 1989.

Dr. Magee has published articles on leukemia, lymphoma, chemotherapy, and peripheral stem cell transplantation. He is a former president of the Nashville Davidson County Unit of the American Cancer Society. He and his wife celebrated their twentieth anniversary in 1997, and they have two sons. He has served as an elder at Westminster Presbyterian Church and at East Brentwood Presbyterian Church. He is assistant scoutmaster for Troop 5, Boy Scouts of America in Brentwood and head coach for his sons' baseball teams.

Karl M. Rogers, M.D., is a native of the American Virgin Islands, where he completed his undergraduate work. He subsequently received his M.P.H. degree from the University of Pittsburgh and, in 1987, his M.D. degree from Rush Medical School in Chicago. His medical oncology training was at Vanderbilt. He is board certified in internal medicine and medical oncology. He is active in the American Cancer Society and the Nashville Oncology Society. He and his wife are members of the First Seventh Day Adventist Church of Nashville and are proud parents of four daughters.

Ken W. Wyman, M.D., is a native of western Kentucky. He earned his bachelor of science degree at Murray State University, in Bowling Green and, in 1990, his M.D. degree from the University of Louisville School of Medicine. He did his medical oncology training at Vanderbilt. He is board certified in internal medicine and medical oncology. His interests outside of medicine include music and travel.

Midstate Oncology and Hematology has been innovative in several areas locally. It was a leader in the outpatient administration of cisplatin and paclitaxel, the treatment of thrombophlebitis as an outpatient with low molecular weight heparin, and the use of a genetic blood test instead of a liver biopsy to diagnose hereditary hemochromatosis.

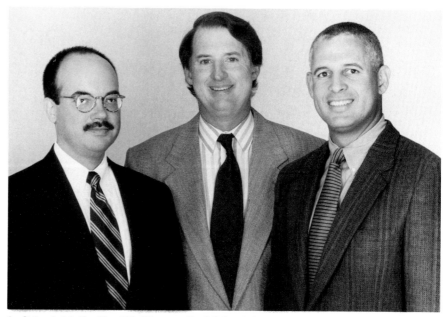

Left to right: Dr. Ken W. Wyman, Dr. Michael J. Magee, and Dr. Karl M.Rogers.

MID-TENNESSEE NEONATOLOGY ASSOCIATES, P.C.

"To take care of small, sick babies—and their mothers and fathers and families—requires passion," says Dr. M. Sami Ismail. "If we did not love this work, we could not do it."

He and five colleagues at Mid-Tennessee Neonatology deal with extreme cases of life-threatening illness among the smallest patients, newborns. "Something can go wrong at any time," Dr. Ismail points out. "We have to be constantly here. These problems we deal with are not something we can tell a nurse over the phone how to handle."

A native of Syria, Dr. Ismail earned his M.D. degree from the Aleppo University in 1977. His postgraduate training included a residency in pediatrics at Wilmington (Delaware) Medical Center and a fellowship in neonatology at the Medical College of Virginia in Richmond. Since coming to Nashville in November, 1989, he has been director of newborn services at Columbia, Centennial Women's Hospital, and served, at various times, on the neonatology staffs at Southern Hills Medical Center, Summit Medical Center, Hendersonville Hospital, Nashville Memorial Hospital, and Metropolitan General Hospital. Among Dr. Ismail's research interests is the significance and application to modern times of the ancient medicine of Arabia.

Dr. Susan Beverin Campbell earned her M.D. at Thomas Jefferson University Medical School in 1973. She did residences in family practice and pediatrics at the Wilmington (Delaware) Medical Center and a fellowship in neonatology at the Milton S. Hershey Medical Center. She holds specialty certification in pediatrics and neonatal-perinatal medicine.

Since 1986 Dr. Campbell has been director of neonatology at Southern Hills Medical Center. From 1989 to the present she has held the same post at Summit Medical Center. She currently serves as a neonatologist at Hendersonville Hospital, Nashville Memorial, Metropolitan General Hospital, and holds faculty appointments at Vanderbilt University Medical Center and the University of Mississippi Medical Center.

Dr. Eric Scott Palmer earned the M.D. degree at the Temple University School of Medicine and did a pediatric internship and residency at the University of Florida's Shands Hospital. He is currently pursuing a fellowship in neonatal medicine at the Vanderbilt University Medical Center. He is board certified by the American Board of Pediatrics.

Dr. Hadeer Noori Karmo received his doctorate in medicine from the Spartan Health Science University, St. Lucia, West Indies. He did residency training at Meharry Medical College and Vanderbilt University, then completed fellowships in neonatology at Vanderbilt, and Henry Ford Hospital, Detroit. He is a diplomate of the American Academy of Pediatrics.

Dr. Anna Arrington Draughn received her medical degree from the Medical College of Georgia in Augusta. She subsequently did her internship and residency training in pediatrics there. She is board certified by the American Board of Pediatrics, is a Fellow of the American Academy of Pediatrics, and holds certifications from the Neonatal Resuscitation Program.

Dr. Sarah Emily Hassell received her M.D. degree from the Medical University of South Carolina in Charleston. She completed an internship and residency in pediatrics at Vanderbilt University Medical Center. She is board certified by the American Board of Pediatrics and holds additional credentials in her specialty from the sub-board for neonatal-perinatal medicine and the neonatal resuscitation program.

James O. Miller, Jr., M.D.

"I never really thought of any other career choice" except medicine, says Madison obstetrician and gynecologist James Miller. Other family members who have pursued the same calling included an uncle, Morris Ferguson, M.D., who was a family practitioner in Lebanon for 40 years; a great uncle, Pete Clark, M.D., who founded a hospital in McMinnville; and a younger brother, Thomas Miller, M.D., who is an internist.

Dr. James Miller is an alumnus of the University of Tennessee Medical School. Following a residency at Vanderbilt, he opened his private practice on July 1, 1974.

In the last 20 years, according to Dr. Miller, the obstetrician-gynecologist has become the primary care physician for an increasing percentage of women. "We are often a woman's principal source of medical care and, in some instances, her only regular medical contact.

"It behooves us to reinforce good health habits, such as regular breast examinations, periodic cervical cytology sampling, family planning, preconceptual counseling, nutrition, and exercise. By strongly emphasizing prenatal care, childbirth education, and a family-centered approach to maternity care, the obstetrician-gynecologist can play a major role in making childbirth safer and more meaningful."

A devoted family man, Dr. Miller, has been married to Cheryl Miller for more than thirty years and has always practiced near his home. "I wanted my three sons to know who I was," he says. Each of them played baseball and basketball, and Dr. Miller can recall missing only half of one basketball game. He and his wife once calculated that they had attended 294 baseball games in a single season.

All of the sons—Richmond, Brandon, and Brent—went on to play college baseball, and the parents drove or flew to each game. Dr. Miller has also become the proud grandfather of Rachel Miller. Dr. Miller plans on practicing obstetrics and gynecology for at least ten more years in the Madison area.

Marcia A. Montgomery, M.D.

A native of Knoxville, Dr. Montgomery is the first member of her family to become a physician. She graduated from the University of Tennessee in Memphis with a bachelor of science degree in medical technology, then entered medical school there in 1971. After receiving the M.D. degree in 1975, she did an internship in internal medicine at Baptist Hospital, Memphis, followed by a residency in obstetrics and gynecology at the City of Memphis Hospital. She chose this specialty because it availed her an opportunity to take care of healthy patients. Since 1982 she has been board certified in obstetrics and gynecology, and is a fellow of the American College of Obstetrics and Gynecology.

In 1979 she entered private practice as a partner in Women Health Associates, P.C. Since 1987 she has limited her practice to gynecology and problems of infertility. She is currently active in scientific research, being affiliated with Clinical Research Associates, where she performs hormone studies and clinical trials.

Dr. Montgomery holds staff appointments at Baptist Hospital, Centennial Medical Center, and Vanderbilt University Medical Center. A member of the Nashville Academy of Medicine and the Tennessee Medical Association, she also belongs to the American Fertility Society and the American Association of Gynecologic Laparoscopists.

Since she was a resident, Dr. Montgomery has shown Westies. In 1996, one of her dogs received the first place award at Westminster in New York, an honor going to the foremost of the breed in the nation.

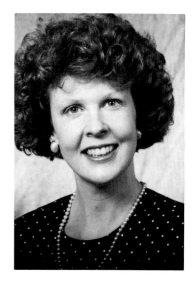

Nashville Ear, Nose, and Throat Clinic

Nashville Ear, Nose, and Throat Clinic offers comprehensive services in adult and pediatric ENT, otology, neurotology, head and neck oncological surgery, skull base surgery, snoring and sleep disorders, rhinology, voice and swallowing disorders, performing arts medicine, audiology and audiovestibular testing, hearing aids, tinnitus management, and laryngology.

The practice has locations in the Centennial and St. Thomas Hospital complexes and at the Cool Springs Medical Center in Franklin, Tennessee. In-office services including laser and radio surgery, rhinopharyngeal stroboscopy, computerized dynamic posturography, auditory brainstem response, electrocochleography, computerized electronystagmography, and programmable digital hearing aids. Inpatient and outpatient surgery services include, but are not limited to, tonsillectomy, adenoidectomy, septoplasty, tymphanoplasty, myringotomy, pediatric eustachian tube placement, cochlear device implantation, removal of tumors of the head and neck, maxillary and nasal sinus endoscopy, stapedectomy, thyroidectomy, and uvulopalatopharyngoplasty.

Physicians in the group are Drs. Mitchell K. Schwaber, Jack A. Coleman, Jr., Stephen A. Mitchell, Jeffrey A. Paffrath, John A. Garside, and James O. Fordice.

Holding the M.D. degree from the University of Cincinnati, Dr. Coleman recalls among pedagogical influences Dr. Charles Aring, a neurologist with whom he spent an intense six weeks studying the human and spiritual side of medicine. Dr. Coleman is a Fellow of the American College of Surgeons. Active in his church, he has also coached martial arts. He is a commander in the U. S. Navy Reserve and maintains a strong interest in military history.

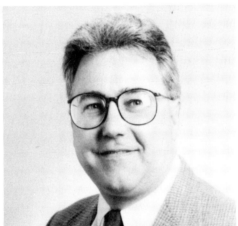

Dr. Jack A. Coleman, Jr.

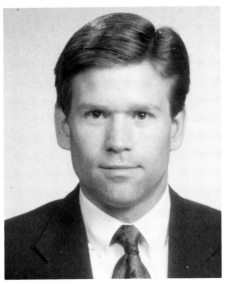

Dr. James O. Fordice

The son of a Presbyterian minister, Dr. Mitchell remembers being exposed as a youngster to problems of human suffering. His great-uncle, Merrick McCarthy, was a prominent otolaryngologist in Cincinnati. Dr. Mitchell received the M.D. degree from the University of Michigan, where he especially recalls his attending, Dr. Nels Olsen. On graduation, Dr. Mitchell served research and clinical clerkships as a naval reserve officer. During his service at the San Diego Naval Hospital, where he was an advisee of Dr. Robert W. Cantrell, Dr. Mitchell developed an interest in caring for professional singers. He eventually became one of the founding members of the Performing Arts Medicine Association. Dr. Mitchell's wife, Karen, is a flautist and flute teacher. Their daughter, Heather, is a film and photography student.

Dr. Fordice considers that his life in medicine follows naturally from "my deep, abiding passion for biology, coupled with an interest in people." He received his medical degree from Baylor, followed by a residency in otolaryngology there, then a fellowship at the University of Texas M.D. Anderson Cancer Center in head and neck surgery. He counts among his mentors his math and physics teacher in high school, Charles Justus; his organic chemistry teacher in college, Dr. Berry; and Dr. Byers one of the faculty at the Anderson Center. Dr. Fordice's wife, Sarina, is also a physician, specializing in radiology, and they are parents of 2 ½ year-old Nicholas.

Dr. John A. Garside holds the M.D. degree from the University of North Carolina School of Medicine and is currently a resident in the department of otolaryngology at the University of Florida School of Medicine. He has also done postgraduate training in general surgery and in head and neck surgery there.

NASHVILLE GASTROINTESTINAL SPECIALISTS, INC.

Nashville Gastrointestinal Specialists comprises Drs. Daniel E. Gremillion, Robert W. Herring, Jr., Allen H. Bailey, and Ronald E. Pruitt. Its facilities include four offices and three ambulatory surgery endoscopy centers. The practice offers state-of-the-art outpatient gastrointestinal and liver services and was among the earliest developers of ambulatory endoscopy centers in Nashville.

Dr. Gremillion completed his undergraduate studies at the University of Notre Dame, then attended medical school at Louisiana State University in New Orleans from 1967-1971. Dr. Gremillion subsequently completed a residency in internal medicine and then a fellowship in gastroenterology at Walter Reed Army Medical Center in Washington, D.C., studying with Dr. H. Worth Boyce, then a leading figure in the evolution of gastrointestinal endoscopy.

Dr. Gremillion has been assistant clinical professor of medicine at the University of Colorado in Denver and the University of Tennessee at Baptist Hospital in Nashville. He has been chief of staff at Southern Hills Medical Center and is currently a member of the board of trustees at Columbia Southern Hills Medical Center. Dr. Gremillion is the senior and founding partner of Nashville Gastrointestinal Specialists, Inc.

Dr. Robert W. Herring, Jr., a native Nashvillian, double-majored in biology and chemistry at Birmingham-Southern College, and received the M.D. degree from the University of Tennessee. He completed his internal medicine residency at Wake Forest University and his gastroenterology and hepatology fellowship at Johns Hopkins University in 1984. Dr. Herring is a Fellow of the American College of Gastroenterology and is board certified in gastroenterology and hepatology. He has been active in organized medicine, serving as president of the Young Physicians Section and chairman of the Governmental Services Committee of the Tennessee Medical Association. Dr. Herring is a board member of the Tennessee chapter of the American College of Physicians and a University of Tennessee faculty member.

Dr. Allan H. Bailey received the M.D. degree from Indiana University Medical School in 1980, then entered the internal medicine residency program at the University of South Florida. Like Dr. Gremillion he came under the influence of Dr. Worth Boyce, director of the division of gastroenterology there. Dr. Bailey pursued a fellowship in gastroenterology at USF from 1983-1985, at a time when many new therapeutic endoscopic procedures were evolving. He is board certified in both internal medicine and gastroenterology and is a Fellow of the American College of Physicians as well as the American College of Gastroenterology.

Dr. Pruitt double majored in chemistry and psychology at the University of North Carolina, Chapel Hill. He earned the M.D. degree from the UNC School of Medicine and completed an internship and residency in internal medicine in 1987 at the University of Alabama School of Medicine, Birmingham, under the direction of his mentor, Basil I. Hirschowitz, M.D., inventor of the flexible fiberoptic endoscope. He completed a fellowship in gastroenterology and hepatology at UAB in 1989. He is board certified in both internal medicine and gastroenterology and is a Fellow of the American College of Physicians as well as the American College of Gastroenterology. Dr. Pruitt is on the faculty of the University of Tennessee School of Medicine. He is president and medical director of Nashville Medical Research Institute.

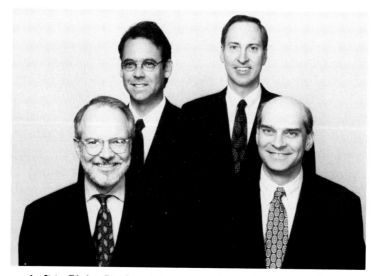

Left to Right: Dr. Gremillion, Dr. Pruitt, Dr. Herring, Dr. Bailey

NASHVILLE PLASTIC SURGERY, PLLC

Nashville Plastic Surgery, PLLC, was founded in 1981 by G. Patrick Maxwell, M.D. Today, with six surgeons, Nashville Plastic Surgery is one of the largest plastic surgery practices in the state. Joining Dr. Maxwell since the founding have been Drs. Jack Fisher, Joseph B. DeLozier III, Greer Ricketson, Mary K. Gingrass, and Bryan D. Oslin.

Founder Patrick Maxwell has been recognized for his innovative surgical techniques, particularly in the fields of breast reconstruction and cosmetic surgery. He was among the pioneers of ultrasonic liposuction in the United States and is an authority on body contouring. He frequently lectures for medical societies and has performed surgical procedures in some 20 countries.

Dr. Maxwell received his medical degree in 1972 from the Vanderbilt University School of Medicine and performed residencies in general and plastic surgery at the Johns Hopkins Hospital in Baltimore. Dr. Maxwell presently serves as medical director of the Institute for Aesthetic and Reconstructive Surgery at Vanderbilt University and as an associate clinical professor in the department of surgery at Meharry Medical College.

Dr. Jack Fisher joined Dr. Maxwell in 1986, having served formerly as an assistant professor of plastic surgery at the Mayo Clinic in Rochester, Minnesota. Dr. Fisher has also been active as a speaker at surgical conferences throughout the world, particularly on the subjects of breast surgery and aesthetic surgery.

Dr. Fisher received his medical degree from Emory University School of Medicine in 1973 and completed his residency in general surgery at George Washington University Medical Center, Washington, D.C. He returned to Emory to perform a residency in plastic surgery. A Fellow in the American College of Surgeons, Dr. Fisher is active in numerous medical societies and is assistant clinical professor in the department of plastic surgery at Vanderbilt University.

Dr. Joseph B. DeLozier, III, became the third member of Nashville Plastic Surgery in 1991. Dr. DeLozier is widely recognized for having operated worldwide on children with facial deformities. He spends two weeks every year in China with Operation Smile International, performing plastic surgery procedures and teaching surgical techniques to Chinese surgeons. He is active in the Tennessee / Kentucky chapter of Operation Smile.

Dr. DeLozier received his medical degree from the University of Tennessee in 1982. Following residencies in general surgery and plastic surgery at Vanderbilt University, he completed a craniofacial fellowship at the University of Pennsylvania and Children's Hospital of Philadelphia.

In 1995 Dr. Mary K. Gingrass became the group's fourth member, and Dr. Greer Ricketson became an associate of the practice.

Dr. Ricketson brought to Nashville Plastic Surgery a wealth of experience and history about the field. He recalls that when he finished his residency in plastic surgery, in 1950, he could name all of his fellow specialists in the country from memory. In those days, only about a quarter of the typical cosmetic surgeon's work was cosmetic in nature. Dr. Ricketson, educated at Vanderbilt, is today largely retired but serves as a valued advisor to younger plastic surgeons.

Dr. Gingrass received her medical degree from the Medical College of Wisconsin in Milwaukee. She completed residencies in general surgery and plastic surgery at Southern Illinois School of Medicine. Dr. Gingrass then completed a fellowship at Nashville Plastic Surgery with an emphasis on aesthetic surgery and breast reconstruction.

Dr. Gingrass was one of the first plastic surgeons in the United States to be trained in the technique of ultrasound-assisted liposuction. She has since taught this technique to other surgeons across the country. Dr. Gingrass serves on the boards of the Tennessee Breast Cancer Coalition and Tennessee Women in Medicine. She is active in legislative efforts concerning women's health issues.

Dr. Bryan D. Oslin joined Nashville Plastic Surgery in 1997. A graduate of Vanderbilt University School of Medicine, he completed his general surgery residency at Vanderbilt in 1994, serving as chief resident in 1993-94. After training in acute and reconstructive burn surgery, Dr. Oslin completed his plastic surgery fellowship at the University of Alabama in Birmingham.

Dr. Oslin's surgical interests today include breast reconstruction, aesthetic facial surgery, body contouring, and microsurgery. He has published in the areas of breast reconstruction and endoscopic facial aesthetic surgery.

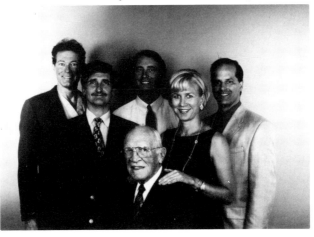

The physicians of Nashville Plastic Surgery, PLLC

NEUROLOGICAL SURGEONS

Neurological Surgeons is a professional corporation comprising board certified neurological surgeons who perform adult neurosurgery at the major hospitals in the metropolitan area of Nashville.

Incorporated in 1983, the group initially consisted of Dr. Everette Howell, Jr., and identical twin brothers Drs. Vaughn and Verne Allen. In 1985, Dr. Timothy Schoettle was asked to join the group. Dr. Gregory Lanford joined in 1991. Dr. Steven Abram became part of the group in 1995. Dr. Scott Standard joined the group in 1997. In February, 1997 Dr. Verne Allen passed away, losing his battle with colon and liver cancer. This was a great loss to the group and to the medical community.

All the physicians in the group went through the Vanderbilt University Medical Center neurosurgery program. Starting with Dr. Schoettle, he and the remaining physicians in the group trained under Dr. Howell and the Drs. Allen. They were carefully chosen to be part of a practice that genuinely cares about people and about giving high quality service. The main goal of the practice has always been to provide the best care possible as well as to be of great service to the community and surrounding areas.

Throughout the years, emphasis has been placed on utilizing newer technological breakthroughs and refining surgical techniques. Surgical procedures for brain tumors and aneurysms, neuro-endovascular procedures, as well as spinal surgery with and without instrumentation are among the special interests of this group.

Neurosurgery is an ever-changing and challenging part of medicine. Neurological Surgeons has a commitment to its continued progress in the future.

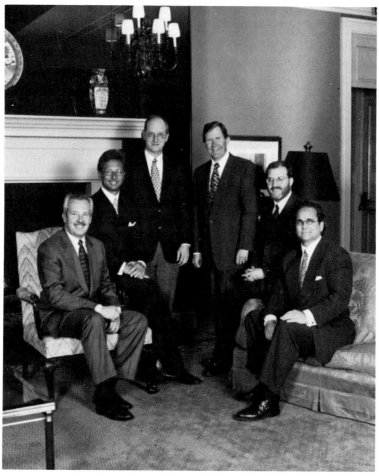

Neurological Surgeon, PC
L to r: Dr. Timothy Schoettle, Dr. Gregory Landord, Dr. Everette Howell, Jr.,
Dr. Vaughan Allen, Dr. Scott Standard, Dr. Steven Abaram

JENNIFER L. OAKLEY, M.D.

In 1900 Dr. Oakley's great grandfather, Thomas J. Ford, received his M.D. from the University of Tennessee Medical School. He then practiced medicine for many years in rural Putnam County, often traveling ten miles or more on horseback to see his patients. His wife died from tuberculosis leaving three daughters, the youngest of whom was Dr. Oakley's grandmother. The children were cared for by local families, and Dr. Ford returned weekly to visit and pay them whatever he had earned. He charged $10 to deliver a baby, but happily accepted an equivalent amount of potatoes, beans, or squash. After his death in 1928, his medical diploma and certificate testifying to his membership in the Paul F. Eve Medicorum Societus passed down through the family. Today, they stand proudly on a shelf in Dr. Oakley's consulting room.

A Candy Striper at age 14, Jennifer Oakley had already determined her career. A college graduate at 19, she entered her grandfather's alma mater in 1977, and received her M.D. degree four years later. She considered specializing in anesthesiology, but after performing her first delivery, she realized that assisting in the birth process was "one of the top things I could ever do. It's a privilege to be part of it." She became a mother herself in 1984, to a son, Blake Oakley Luttrell.

Dr. Oakley completed an internship / residency in obstetrics and gynecology in 1985, and was certified as a fellow of the American Board of Obstetrics and Gynecology in 1987, with recertification in 1995. She names Dr. Bertram Buxton, Professor of Obstetrics and Gynecology, as one of the outstanding physicians who has influenced her. "He epitomized kindness, intelligence, and love for patients."

In 1985 Dr. Oakley entered private practice at the Jackson Clinic in Dickson, then in 1987 returned to her home town of Nashville. She limits her practice to gynecology, now concentrating on the non-childbearing needs of women of all ages.

In the century since Dr. Ford's day, new opportunities are available to physicians, and Dr. Oakley has enjoyed many of them. She taught as a clinical instructor at Vanderbilt University Medical Center and has lectured before physicians, operating room staffs, and the public. She is on the active medical staffs of St. Thomas, Baptist, and Centennial Medical Centers, and from 1994 through 1996 served on the Centennial Medical Center Board of Trustees.

In 1992 Dr. Oakley and eleven colleagues founded Tennessee Women in Medicine to promote interest in women's health issues. During her presidency, 1994 to 1996, the group created a scholarship, which goes each year to a deserving female medical student. The organization has also worked with Tennessee legislators to bring about better laws affecting health care for women, including those applicable to breast cancer reconstructive surgery.

As a member of the International Society of Gynecologic Endoscopy, Dr. Oakley enjoys the privilege of sharing new minimally invasive surgical techniques, protocols, and information worldwide. In the view of Dr. Oakley, these techniques have allowed patients to "suffer less pain, less complications, shorter hospital stays, and less loss of income."

Although new opportunities exist for physicians, one remains the same as in Dr. Ford's era, the "opportunity to serve." Dr. Oakley insists that her "best accolades are my patients and my children," her son and those whom she delivered.

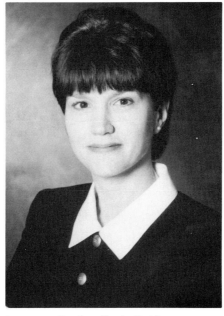
Dr. Jennifer L. Oakley

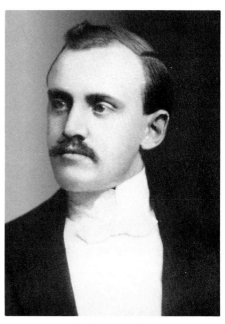
Dr. Thomas Ford

PAGE-CAMPBELL CARDIOLOGY GROUP

The Page-Campbell Cardiology Group practices cardiovascular medicine with offices at St. Thomas Hospital and Vanderbilt University Medical Center in Nashville, Middle Tennessee Medical Center in Murfreesboro, and Cookeville Regional Medical Center in Cookeville. The group comprises 21 physicians who are board certified in cardiovascular diseases, including two physicians who are board certified in clinical cardiac electrophysiology.

Dr. Harry L. Page started the group in 1968 after founding the only cardiac catheterization laboratory in Nashville outside the medical schools. Dr. W. Barton Campbell joined Dr. Page in 1970, and in 1974, Cardiology Consultants, P.C. was incorporated. The name was changed in 1995 to honor the two founding partners. In 1994 Dr. Page was elected Governor of the American College of Cardiology for Tennessee.

Listing the 'firsts' performed or introduced locally by Drs. Page and Campbell would exceed the scope of this profile and, in any event, are well-known to their colleagues. Their pioneering efforts have been continued by subsequent members of the practice with intracoronary laser angioplasty, transfemoral aortic valvuloplasty, intracoronary stenting, intracoronary ultrasound, transesophageal ultrasound, transradical percutaneous coronary angioplast (PTCA), and outpatient PTCA.

In Nashville the group has helped develop outpatient coronary angiography, the use of thrombolytic therapy for acute myocardial infarction, primary PTCA for acute myocardial infarction, and office cardioversion for atrial fibrillation. In 1988, Page-Campbell Cardiology Group founded the clinical electrophysiology laboratory at St. Thomas Hospital. No other such facility then existed in Middle Tennessee outside of academic medical centers.

Page-Campbell Cardiology Group established the cardiac catheterization laboratory at Middle Tennessee Medical Center in Murfreesboro and has guided the growth of cardiac services at that hospital. In 1997, Page-Campbell Cardiology and Upper Cumberland Cardiology of Cookeville merged their practices. The Cookeville physicians have continued to provide cardiology leadership at Cookeville Regional Medical Center as it has expanded its scope of cardiovascular services.

As the practice has grown, the emphasis had been on maintaining a high level of expertise through sub-specialization within the field of cardiovascular medicine. The group has recruited physicians with specialized training and certification in clinical cardiac electrophysiology and cardiac pacing, nuclear cardiology (including PET imaging), echocardiography, and interventional cardiology.

The physicians of Page-Campbell have a long tradition of involvement in teaching and research. Collaborative projects with Vanderbilt University Medical Center and Meharry Medical College have included teaching of students, house staff, and cardiology fellows. Page-Campbell physicians have worked with colleagues in the Vanderbilt Cardiology Division to enroll patients in several large national clinical trials.

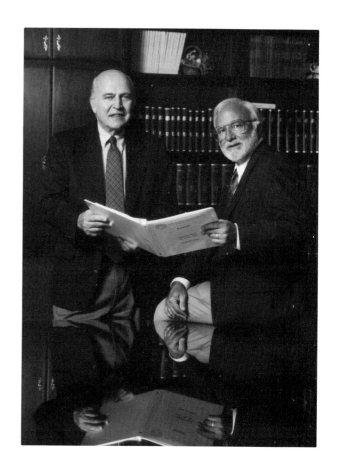

Over the past 30 years, the Page-Campbell Cardiology Group has witnessed dramatic changes in the practice of cardiovascular medicine. As we enter the next century, we will continue to provide high quality medical care while developing treatment strategies that insure efficient utilization of medical resources. We believe that accountability for treatment outcomes and appropriate utilization of resources, along with a commitment to high quality of practice, will result in lower-cost medical care. It is our hope that in future years we can continue to share with our medical communities the professional rewards we have enjoyed in the form of continued improvement in patient care and the education of the physicians who will eventually take our places.

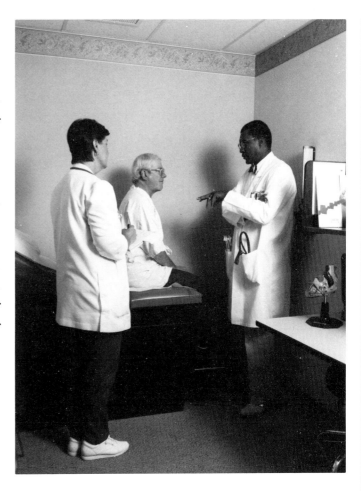

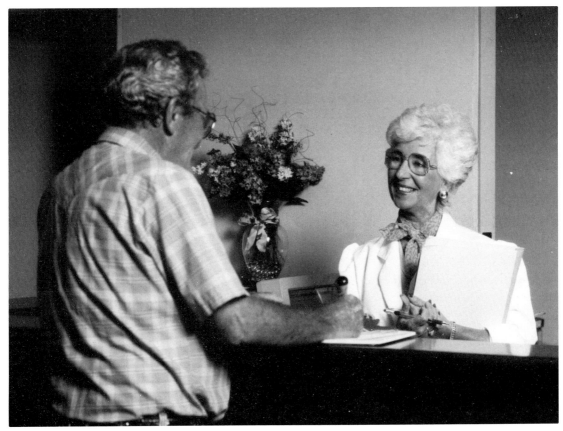

RADIOLOGY CONSULTANTS, INC.

The group began in 1954 when Dr. Ingram and Dr. Hamilton opened an office in the West End Building. Later, they built an office at 2119 Hayes Street.

By 1961 its largest site was a one-room department at Park Vista Convalescent Center. Other clients of years past include Miller Clinic, Park View Hospital, Tennessee Christian Medical Center, Williamson County Hospital, and health care facilities at Columbia, Lewisburg, Portland, and Bowling Green, Kentucky.

Currently the group covers multiple sites, most affiliated with Columbia. Its principal location is a multispecialty department within Centennial Medical Center. Other sites on the Centennial campus include The Women's Hospital, Women's Breast Center, and Medical Plaza Diagnostic Center. The Women's Breast Center provides evaluation and diagnosis of lesions in the breast using mammography, dedicated breast ultrasound, and stereotactic breast biopsy. Medical Plaza Diagnostic Center specializes in gynecological and obstetric ultrasound, including high-risk pregnancy.

Over the years Radiology Consultants has matured into a subspecialty and multidimensional practice. Its affiliated physicians have fellowship training and teaching experience in contemporary subspecialties of radiology as well as expertise in the newest technological advances in the field. It possesses state-of-the-art equipment, enabling it to achieve leading-edge techniques and radiographic protocols in magnetic resonance imaging, CT, ultrasound, nuclear medicine, and other areas.

In 1987 Radiology Consultants opened an outpatient imaging center called Quantum at 2018 Murphy Avenue. Here the group provides MRI, CT, and general radiology services.

In February 1996 the practice began offering teleradiology services using a wide-area network with T1 lines. It now provides all radiology services to Trinity Hospital in Erin and subspecialty expertise to Crockett Hospital in Lawrenceburg.

Radiology Consultants currently comprises Drs. William S. Keane (interventional radiology), Charles T. Faulkner (general and women's imaging), Frank B. Glascock (general and women's imaging), Robert S. Francis (general and women's imaging), Edward M. Priest (interventional radiology), Charles L. Robinette, Jr. (neuroradiology), James D. Green (general, MRI, and CT), Glynis Sacks (ultrasound), Alice Hinton (women's imaging), Michael E. Edwards (interventional radiology), Scott A. Montesi (chest and general), Christopher C. Ng (CT and MRI), Kurt V. Berger (CT and MRI), Brian L. Berger (neuro and neurointerventional radiology), Robert L. Bell (nuclear medicine), Scott D. Gray (musculoskeletal radiology), Edward B. Schmidt (general), Joseph B. Cornett (neuro and neurointerventional radiology), James A. Martin (general), and Stephanie P. Y.. Yen (nuclear medicine / general). Retired or deceased members include Drs. Ingram, Hamilton, Linn, Farrar, Silbert, and Smith.

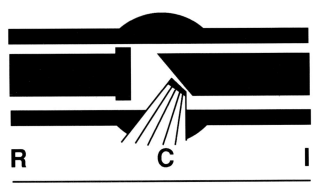

RADIOLOGY CONSULTANTS, INC.

WILLIAM B. RALPH, JR., M.D.

A native of Sumner County, Dr. Ralph grew up on his parents' farm there. While still in elementary school, he began looking forward to one day studying and practicing medicine. "I always had great respect for physicians," Dr. Ralph remembers. He, his father, and mother held the family pediatrician, Dr. Jimmy Overall, in particularly high regard.

As a teenager, the youngster became a patient of Dr. Clarence Thomas, Sr., head of the department of allergy at Vanderbilt, and remained one through undergraduate and medical school years there. "Dr. Thomas was the most thorough physician I've ever known," Dr. Ralph added. "He didn't miss a thing." From his years in medical school, Dr. Ralph also recalls with admiration Dr. John Shapiro, head of the department of pathology. "He was a highly stimulating

teacher, and there has never been one more fair to students."

As Dr. Ralph was finishing his fellowship training at Duke, Dr. Thomas invited him to return to Nashville and form a joint practice. They became partners in 1974.

Dr. Ralph's professional service includes the presidency of the Middle Tennessee Lung Association and the Southeast Allergy Association. In civic affairs he was a member of the Leadership Nashville Class of 1985, and he serves as an elder of the Westminster Presbyterian Church. He and his wife, Elizabeth, have five children: Will, III; twins Lucy and Rebecca, daughter Claiborne, and Molly. The Ralph family (those big enough to hold a racket, at least) are avid tennis players, and they have a block of seats at Vanderbilt basketball games.

ANTHONY E. D. TRABUE, M.D.

Dr. Trabue traces his family line back through ten generations of Middle Tennesseans. Among these forebears was Dr. Charles Trabue, a surgeon and the first chief of staff at Baptist Hospital after it was reorganized from Protestant Hospital.

Early in his life Anthony Trabue knew what his vocation would be. From age 16, he worked in hospitals, mopping floors, moving patients, shooting x-rays, and assisting in surgery. He majored in European history at Vanderbilt "because I knew I was going to be immersed in science."

Entering Vanderbilt Medical School in 1971, he followed his training with an internship in general surgery and a fellowship in obstetrics and gynecology. He recalls Dr. Jack Davies , an anatomy professor, "a great scientist and kind man." He adds, "Dr. Thomas Brittingham was everyone's role model in the clinical years."

Dr. Trabue opened a private practice in obstetrics and gynecology in 1979 and has been a solo practitioner since 1984. In 1983 he was elected the outstanding clinical in-

structor by the Vanderbilt House Staff, receiving the Everett Clayton Award. He is a fellow of the American College of Obstetrics and Gynecology.

His professional service has been concentrated at Centennial Medical Center, where he served as either chairman or vice chairman of the ob-gyn department from 1996 to 1998. For four years he has been a member of the board of trust.

Dr. Anthony is married to Dr. Ramona, a retired obstetrician, and they are the parents of Christopher, Suzanna, William, Mary Elizabeth, Joanna, Tom, and Sam. Dr. Trabue adds, "I have dedicated my life to my God, my family, and the women and unborn children of Middle Tennessee, the United States, and the world."

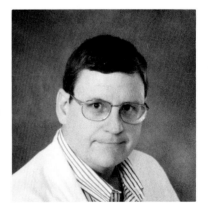

STEWART SHOFNER, M.D.

When asked why he chose his speciality, ophthalmologist Stewart Shofner exclaims, "I delight in helping people see clearly!"

Dr. Shofner grew up on a farm in Shelbyville, the son of Kathleen King Shofner and Brigadier General Austin C. Shofner, a decorated Marine hero of World War II. "On our parents' farm we would do a hard day's work, then at the end, we could see a new fence up, or an acre cleared—real results."

Young Shofner did his undergraduate years at Harvard, studying with, among others, George Wald, the Nobel laureate. He recalls Dr. Wald's course in first-year biology and his classic half-hour lecture that drew together basic principles of biology and physics. "Dr. Wald inspired me to go into medicine," Dr. Shofner recalls. He entered medical school at the University of Virginia, where he was drawn to neurology. "I liked that subject because after thoroughly examining the patient, you can have a 99 percent confidence level about what the lesion is and where it is." But he was not impressed with the success rate of neurosurgery.

Then one day on rounds in the neurology ward, Dr. Shofner followed a patient with an flame hemorrhage to the ophthalmology wing. "When the patient's eyes had been dilated, I could look into the back of the eye and see the problem."

His interest piqued, he completed an ophthalmology residency at Yale, then did a Louisiana State University Corneal Fellowship. There he received specialty training in corneal transplant surgery, corneal and external diseases, anterior segment reconstructive surgery, and refractive surgery. As a corneal fellow, Dr. Shofner surgically assisted in the treatment of normally sighted myopic patients utilizing Excimer laser photorefractive keratectomy.

Corneal transplants are another way that Dr. Shofner practices the hands-on medicine that he loves. "The success rate of a corneal transplant staying in without a graft rejection is 95 percent. It's lower for more difficult cases, of course, but that's a good point to start from.

"Cataract surgery allows the surgeon to make a major change in an individual's life," he says. "Being able to restore sight to people who have not had sight for a long time can be extremely gratifying."

Dr. Shofner is board certified by the American Board of Opthalmology and is a fellow of the American Academy of Ophthalmology. He has been on the clinical faculty of the James H. Quillen College of Medicine and has contributed papers to journals of ophthalmology and corneal research.

Dr. Shofner is married to Dr. Ann Kalisz, an internist, and they have three children, Robert Stewart, Alyssa Ann, and Andrew Conner. Dr. Shofner greatly enjoys sculpting, an art that, like surgery, requires manual dexterity. Describing himself as a "frustrated artist," Dr. Shofner particularly enjoys working in wood and in alabaster.

Three siblings reside in Middle Tennessee. Wes is an attorney and Martin is an architect; both practice in Nashville. Michael is in the financial business with their father in Shelbyville, where Shofner ancestors founded the first Lutheran church west of the Appalachian Mountains in the early 1800s.

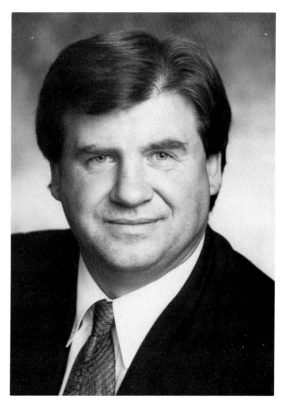

BUNTWAL N. SOMAYAJI, M.D.

"By age 15, even before I knew what life was all about, I had to make a choice about my vocation," says Dr. Somayaji. The choice he made has taken him from his native city of Mangalore in southern India, to the British isles, and, finally, to Nashville.

After earning his medical degree at Madras Medical College, Dr. Somayaji performed his residency in New Delhi before relocating to England. In 1967 he earned the M.R.C.P. (London), a distinction that allowed him to practice anywhere in the British Commonwealth.

His special interest in gastroenterology evolved during his training and led him to the United States in 1968 to gain experience in endoscopy. He won fellowships in gastroenterology at the M. D. Anderson Hospital at the University of Texas, Houston. In January, 1970, Dr. Somayaji accepted an offer from Meharry Medical College to organize a division of gastroenterology and set up an endoscopy laboratory. After four years there, he entered into private practice at Baptist and Memorial Hospitals. He retains appointment as the director of Meharry's division of gastroenterology and is chief of gastroenterology at Metropolitan Nashville General Hospital. He took an active part in developing gastroenterology laboratories at Baptist, Memorial, and Hubbard Hospitals.

Dr. Somayaji has given back to his adopted home in numerous ways. From 1980 to 1994 he served as founding chairman of the board of trustees of Sri Ganesha Temple and Hindu Cultural Center of Tennessee. The group was formed in October, 1980. The Sri Ganesha Temple affords a place of worship for 6,000-7,000 families from Tennessee and seven surrounding states. The Center is also open to persons from the community at large interested in exploring more about the Hindu traditions and philosophy.

Since 1991 Dr. Somayaji has served as a national trustee of the National Conference for Community and Justice (formerly known as the National Conference of Christians and Jews). He says, "Lots of problems in our city and in our society stem from the fact that people don't understand each other. I became involved in the National Conference to fight bias, bigotry, and racism and to promote understanding among all races, religions, and cultures. We do that through advocacy, conflict resolution, and education." For his work in this field Dr. Somayaji received the Conference's 1997 Human Relations Award. He was a member of Leadership Nashville's Class of 1997-98.

Dr. Somayaji is a diplomate of the American Board of Internal Medicine, with a subspecialty in gastroenterology. He is also a fellow of the American College of Physicians. He has served on several committees of the Nashville Academy of Medicine including program and credentials, and co-chaired the medico-legal panel from 1988-92.

In addition to practicing and teaching gastroenterology, Dr. Somayaji is involved in several philanthropic enterprises in India, mainly educational institutions.

"I hope that my varied experiences can contribute to improving the quality of life for everybody with whom I come in contact," Dr. Somayaji says.

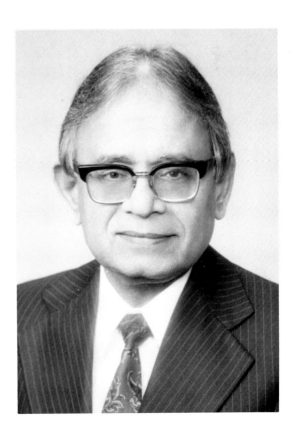

St. Thomas Hospital

As St. Thomas celebrated its centennial anniversary in April, 1998, it consistently ranks among the top five cardiac centers in the nation performing more than 2,300 open heart procedures annually. St. Thomas Hospital is part of a rich and caring service heritage.

Named for Nashville's Bishop Thomas Byrne's patron saint, St. Thomas the Apostle, the hospital originated with the vision of the Daughter of Charity, an order of Catholic nuns/religious women as a twenty-bed sanitarium on Hayes Street. First founded in Paris, France in 1633, by St. Vincent de Paul and St. Louise de Marillae, the nuns organized and trained young peasant women to care for the less fortunate and later expanded their mission to educating children and caring for the sick in hospitals and on battlefields.

As pioneers of modern social services, the Daughters organized European orphanages, homes for the aged and for unwed mothers, soup kitchens, and hotels for beggars. They also were early advocates for prisoners' reforms and war

relief. Their charity extended across the Atlantic when the Daughters of Charity of St. Vincent de Paul favorably replied to Bishop Byrne's request to build a hospital in Nashville. In January, 1898, the Corporation of St. Joseph officially purchased and registered the property after $20,000 came to Bishop Byrne. What once was a Hayes Street mansion became a 26-bed, 16-room hospital that included a kitchen, a chapel, and living quarters for the five Sisters. A $30,000 note was secured to help the Sisters with renovation costs.

The staff of four nurses and a housekeeper found the space more than adequate; however, patronage for the new hospital was slow in coming. Despite financial hardships resulting in the Sister's selling chandeliers from the chapel for $250 to pay for maintenance, the hospital was filled with 33 patients in 1899. It was in this year that St. Thomas appeared in the records of the state medical association for the first time. Also during this time the St. Thomas and staff

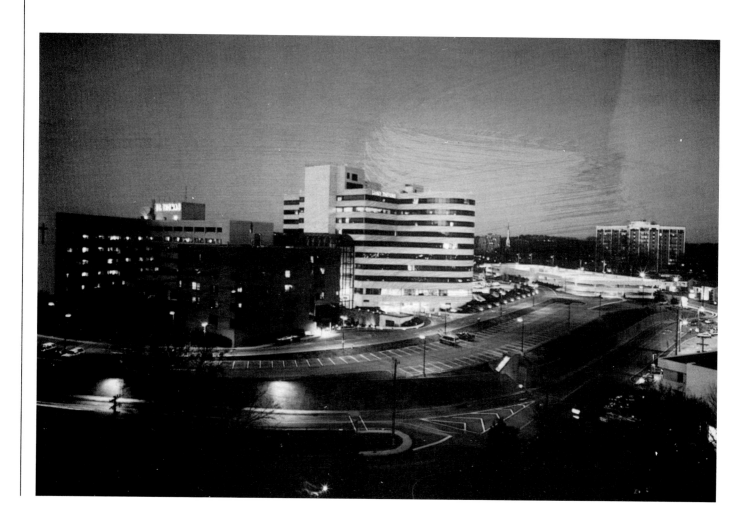

nursed to recovery veterans of the Civil War and the Spanish-American War. Many of the Daughters themselves became ill with yellow fever and malaria, and four did not survive.

At the turn of the century, the Sisters recognized the need for additional space required by major medical developments. The grand opening of the new, 150-bed facility took place on January 29, 1902. To provide a consistent and competent nursing staff, the St. Thomas School of Nursing opened in April of 1902. St. Thomas was incorporated on December 2, 1905, thus changing the financial picture for the hospital. As a nonprofit organization, any gains from continued operation were placed back into improved services and facilities. The hospital census showed 110 patients in December of 1910, 1,873 patients between the years 1911 and 1912, and 2,648 during 1915. In 1914 the hospital approved an internship program that brought young qualified physicians to the staff.

The six-story St. Thomas of the 1930s and 40s held beds for 225 patients, facilitated care for debilitating diseases such as polio and rheumatic fever, accommodated the less fortunate during the Great Depression and compensated for staff lost to World War II. In spite of what seemed grave limitations for the medical community, St. Thomas evidenced a remarkable 6,594 admitted patients, 4,145 operations performed, 5,921 patients cured or improved, and 827 live births during 1940.

The times saw the introduction of new drugs and procedures. For example penicillin and streptomycin proved effective in treating infectious bacterial diseases rendering the TB ward a service of the past. Between 1946 and 1950 diseases at St. Thomas were reduced by 75% as a result.

Amidst the social upheaval and the advent of more specialized and sophisticated health care methodologies of the 1960s, St. Thomas managed to comfortably adapt and to competently serve the growing area. St. Thomas facilitated Nashville racial integration when an African-American obstetrical nurse asked to deliver her own baby there. A cardiac intensive care unit added ten beds with highly monitored care for surgical and medical patients. Vascular surgery became a reality in 1967. In 1966, St. Thomas performed its first transabdominal intrauterine fetal transfusion. On Christmas Day, 1969, the hospital inaugurated family centered maternity care with unlimited visiting hours for fathers. Classes for expectant parents were introduced at this time as well.

In the late 1960s a new hospital on a 28-acre tract of land on Harding Road was proposed. Plans called for site work to begin in 1971, and the new building was completed in 1974 at a total cost of $21 million. On Saturday, December 21st, local volunteers and the Fort Knox Army Reserve Medical Personnel helped transport patients and equipment. The patients of St. Thomas were settled into their new rooms in time for lunch. In addition to the 410 beds, St. Thomas added 25 single patient rooms to create a mental health unit. Although a Catholic oriented facility, St. Thomas addressed the need to represent the ecumenical patient base in 1976 by welcoming four United Methodist chaplaincy interns to the pastoral care department.

Today St. Thomas is one of the nation's outstanding regional tertiary hospitals and the anchor of St. Thomas Health Services. The 571-bed acute and medical, surgical, and sub-acute care facility provides health care services for a population of more than two million in northern Alabama, southwestern Kentucky, and middle Tennessee. St. Thomas had become a cardiac care leader in the 1990s with over 80% of cardiac patients from outside Davidson County. Upon performing more than 20,000 open heart surgeries, St. Thomas was recognized as third in the nation in volume of open heart procedures for Medicare patients in 1992. By 1995, 129 patients had received heart transplants. While guided by the Daughters of Charity mission to make a positive difference in the lives and health status of both individuals and communities, St. Thomas provided a yearly average of $36 million in charity care and community benefit programs between 1993 and 1997. St. Thomas is dedicated to providing health care that is spiritually centered, accessible, and affordable.

The staff of St. Thomas and its entities share in the rich heritage of the early health care pioneers and continue in their own way to fulfill the mission to serve the sick, needy, and dying with an abiding love and respect for all of God's children.

Dan M. Spengler, M.D.

Given the fact that his parents, Harold and Wilhelmina Spengler, emphasized the value of education, Dan Spengler was bound toward a professional goal early in life. His first interest was engineering, and he earned a scholarship in engineering to Baldwin-Wallace College in Berea, Ohio, across the state from his native town of Defiance.

In his undergraduate years, he found that he liked the biological sciences, and he recalled a family friend back home, Dr. Jim Cameron, a compassionate surgeon who was an alumnus of the University of Michigan Medical School. Graduating with honors in chemistry, the young man applied to and was accepted at Dr. Cameron's alma mater. There he had the privilege of studying with Drs. Cameron Haight, one of the nation's leading thoracic surgeons; neurosurgeon Edgar Kahn—who supposedly was the model for Dr. Robert Merrick in Lloyd C. Douglas's immensely popular novel *Magnificent Obsession*—and Bill Smith, chief of orthopaedics.

Dr. Spengler graduated in 1966 and entered on an internship at King County Hospital in Seattle. Thereafter he returned to the University of Michigan Medical Center for residencies in general surgery and in orthopaedics. As a surgeon with the United States Air Force, he served a tour of duty at Milphap Hospital in Phan Rang, South Viet Nam, and in 1970 was awarded the Bronze Star for meritorious service.

In 1974 Dr. Spengler completed a fellowship in biomechanics at Case Western Reserve. Since that time he has remained in academic medicine. After 10 years at the University of Washington, he accepted the post of professor and chairman of the department of orthopaedics and rehabilitation at Vanderbilt, which he holds today. He is also chief of orthopaedics and rehabilitation at the Vanderbilt University Medical Center and a consultant at the Veteran's Administration Hospital.

In addition to being editor of the *Journal of Spine Disorders* and a reviewer and consultant to the editorial boards of other scientific publications, Dr. Spengler has himself published widely. His books include *Low Back Pain: Evaluation and Management*; *Orthopaedic Practice* (with Philip M. Yeoman); and a volume co-edited with several others, *Instrumented Fusion of the Degenerative Lumbar Spine*. Dr. Spengler has served as a visiting lecturer and professor at schools of medicine here and abroad, and is a member of

various professional organizations. These memberships include the Nashville Academy of Medicine, the Nashville Surgical Society, and the Tennessee Medical Association. Nationally, his peers elected him president of the American Board of Orthopaedic Surgery, in which post he served from 1993-94.

Dr. Spengler has won grants supporting investigations in bone strength, osteoporosis, low back pain, and lumbar spine research, among other specialized subjects. On his office wall he displays the VOLVO Award for Basic Science Research that he received in 1990, awarded for the research that he and three other researchers made into physiological conditions and mechanical properties in intervertebral discs. The next year he was honored with a Kappa Delta award for his longitudinal study of industrial low back pain, conducted with several colleagues.

The Spengler family includes wife Cynthia, daughter Christie, and son Craig. They enjoy skiing, hiking, and golf.

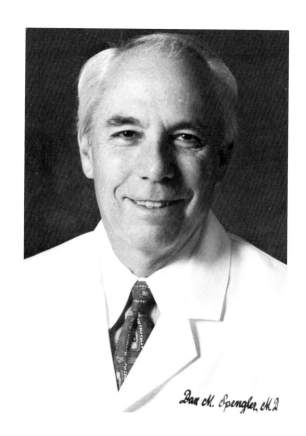

Dan M. Spengler, M.D.

TENNESSEE ONCOLOGY, PLLC

Tennessee Oncology, PLLC, is a physician-owned medical practice specializing in oncology and hematology. The mission of Tennessee Oncology is to provide excellence through a commitment to patient satisfaction through educational and emotional support; the development of clinical research and innovative treatment protocols; and high-quality, cost-effective patient care. The group consists of 24 Middle Tennessee clinics and 18 practicing physicians.

Nashville Oncology-Hematology, PC, was formed as a solo practice in 1976 by Dr. Stuart Spigel. In 1982 Dr. Charles McKay joined the practice, followed by Dr. Eric Raefsky in 1989. Over the next thirteen years, the practice expanded by merging with and hiring oncologists to form Tennessee Oncology, PLLC.

In 1993 Drs. Anthony Greco and John Hainsworth, formerly of the Vanderbilt Cancer Research and Treatment Center, joined the practice to develop an oncology drug research program. These Phase II and Phase III studies give patients who have not responded to first-line therapies the opportunity to receive the most up-to-date drugs and innovative medical treatments available. Of the numerous ongoing research studies, a major focus is directed toward breast and lung cancer and carcinoma of unknown primary origin.

Drs. Anthony Meluch, from the University of Alabama, Birmingham, and Dana Thompson, of the Vanderbilt University Medical Center, joined the practice in 1993. In 1995 the private practice of Drs. Michael Kuzur, Fernando Miranda, and Patricia Bihl, merged with the group, adding the former's existing Nashville Memorial Hospital patient base. At this time, the company was reorganized as Tennessee Oncology.

Subsequent to the merger in 1996, Drs. Nancy Peacock, formerly of South Texas Oncology-Hematology Associates in San Antonio; Jeffrey Patton, formerly of the Lewis-Gale Clinic in Salem, Virginia; and Mary Rachel Faris, a practicing oncologist with the U. S. Army, joined the group.

In 1997 Dr. Howard (Skip) Burris, formerly Director of the University of Texas Health Sciences Clinical Research Program, joined Tennessee Oncology to conduct development of new investigational agents through Phase I (first-time human testing) and Phase II research trials.

Also joining Tennessee Oncology in 1997 was Dr. John Barton, formerly of the Hematology-Oncology Associates Clinic in Harrisburg, Virginia. In 1998 the Tullahoma and Winchester practice of Dr. Mainuddin Ahmed was merged into the group. Also joining the practice that year were Drs. Mitchell Toomey from St. Mary's Regional Cancer Center in Huntington, West Virginia, and Victor Gian, from the University of Florida Oncology Division in Gainesville.

The emphasis of Tennessee Oncology is based on the belief that every patient deserves the very best oncology care available through an integrated network system of outpatient services. These services include the standard treatment modalities of chemotherapy and radiation, as well as treatment through innovative research protocols. Tennessee Oncology is committed to continuing its vision for the latest treatment advancements and premier patient care in the specialties of oncology and hematology.

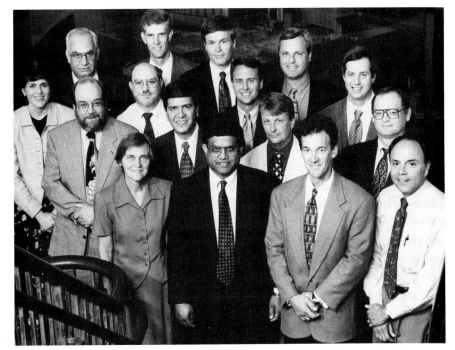

Back Row, l-r: Michel Kuzur, M.D., John Barton, M.D., John D. Hainsworth, M.D., Howard "Skip" Burris, M.D. **Next Row:** Nancy Peacock, M.D., Eric L. Raefsky, M.D., Jeffrey F. Patton, M.D., Charles E. McKay, M.D. **Next Row:** Anthony Greco, M.D., Fernando Miranca, M.D., Dana Thompson, M.D., Victor Gian, M.D. **Front Row:** Patricia Bihl, M.D., Mainuddin Ahmed, M.D., Anthony Meluch, M.D., Stuart Spigel, M.D.

TENNESSEE CHRISTIAN MEDICAL CENTER

Tennessee Christian Medical Center (TCMC), is a 361-bed hospital with a 350-member medical staff and a team of 1,000 professional employees. Serving approximately 35,000 patients annually by providing out-patient and in-patient acute care on two campuses, TCMC's main facility is located in Madison with a satellite facility in Portland, Tennessee. The founders of the hospital realized that total health depends on a balance of physical, mental, psychological, and spiritual well-being, a philosophy embodied in the Seventh-day Adventist healthcare system for over a century. TCMC, like Adventist Health System (AHS), reflects a tradition of promoting the integration of scientific treatment of disease and prevention of disease using educational tools that originated over a century ago in Battle Creek, Michigan.

TCMC is part of a rich and beautiful heritage beginning during a two-fold mission in June, 1904 when a missionary steamboat, "The Morning Star," anchored amid the Cumberland River on the outskirts of Madison, Tennessee. Among the passengers were James Edson White, Ellen White, and E. A. Sutherland who chanced observing the Nelson Ferguson Farm off Neely's Bend at Larkin Springs. It was Ellen White who first perceived the land as a perfect place for a sanitarium by confessing that she had seen the land in a vision and that God's will was to settle and establish a school on that very land. James White, Edward A. Sutherland and Percy T. Magan felt that immense, rocky and barren land too much of a financial responsibility, but Mrs. White adamantly refused to deny God's counsel. With the assistance of Elder George I. Butler, president of the southern Union Conference of Seventh-day Adventists, and Elder S. N. Haskell, an evangelistic leader, a legacy of spiritual healthcare began.

This group formed the holding corporation and organization once known as the Nashville Agricultural and Normal Institute, the precursor of Madison College. The Nashville Agricultural and Normal Institute consisted of eleven students and several dilapidated farm buildings on 400 acres purchased by E.A. Sutherland and four other teachers. Sutherland strongly believed that a college education should be made available to any student willing to labor for it. Each student was expected to work for one half to all of his tuition and other academic expenses and would leave the school competent in two or more professions to ensure success. More than three hundred students from thirty-six states and in foreign countries comprised the earliest class. To main-

tain a balance between service and academic requirements, the students were expected to work five hours daily and study five hours. Since Madison accepted students exclusively because they lacked financial means for a college education, their work was credited toward living expenses and tuition. Madison offered a variety of educational opportunities such as nursing, medical work, home economics, and agriculture.

As president of the self-supporting Madison School, Sutherland alongside Professor Magan and Mrs. White, visualized health care integrated with academics. Adventist schools at this time did not operate sanitariums nor did these men have plans for establishing a medical school—but ironically the idea, coupled with church affiliation proved to break the barriers needed to provide better service. Today practically every self-supporting unit in the South considers medical work an essential part of its program.

It was James and Ellen White who laid the foundation of health care for Madison. Due to their own poor health and unsuccessful encounters with medical prescriptions, they took an interest in natural remedies such as sunshine, fresh air and water, exercise, avoidance of smoking and alcohol, and eating nutritious foods low in sugar and fat. They recognized the effectiveness of the Biblical concepts of good health, as written in the creation story, and integrated teaching them to others. Research demonstrates the effectiveness of these methods today. The creation-based lifestyle changes recommended by the Adventist church and Madison Sanitarium a century ago have become common to nearly every healthful diet.

Madison Foods originated in the 1930s as a result of avid student involvement and excellent administrative supervision. They specialized in over two hundred varieties of soybean products and soy milk for infant formula. The students also manufactured brooms, rugs, floor coverings, and photographic prints. Funds raised were routed directly back to the school. In addition to those commodities, the students provided their own maintenance services while learning trades such as plumbing, plastering, carpentry, architecture, steamfitting, and electrical work. The school boasted the finest arboretum and botanical gardens in the state.

Medical care originated when a Nashville businessman seeking health via the value of diet and treatment principles held by the Madison people asked to be admitted as a patient. The end of the porch served as his room since no facilities to accommodate him were available. The first building for the sanitarium, a small kerosene-lighted cottage with an eleven-bed capacity, contained three treatment rooms opening to a porch. A wide board placed atop two wooden sawhorses made an examination table, yet to these humble rooms entered many of Nashville's elite searching for physical and spiritual healing. In 1906 an eight-room cottage was built with another twelve rooms added the next year to accommodate the sick.

By 1914 Sutherland and Magan, convinced that Madison should implement health care services, had secured their medical degrees from a Nashville college. By the 1930s the Madison Rural Sanitarium, as it was then called, grew to eight hundred acres, one hundred rooms, state of the art medical equipment, and fourteen physicians on staff. It earned funds for the college but did not refuse treating charity patients. With the assistance of capable teachers, administrators, and supporters, the school advanced to a high school, to a junior college then an accredited four-year college by 1933. In ten years, forty units patterned after Madison operated throughout the South.

The number of graduates totaled 1,000 at the Golden Anniversary observance in 1954 and of these, 258 entered self-supporting enterprises, 138 became denominational explorers in America, and 51 served foreign services. During these fifty years, 223 faculty members served the institution. The sanitarium, then a 220-bed facility, had trained 500 graduate nurses. A family of 125 workers lived on campus and performed all the tasks connected with the school, sanitarium, farm, and other industries. Forty-three private homes, eleven cabins, and two apartment houses then belonged to the institution. After the 1962 additions, Madison became a 310-bed facility that provided training in professional and licensed practical nursing, anesthesia, medical records, and X-ray technology.

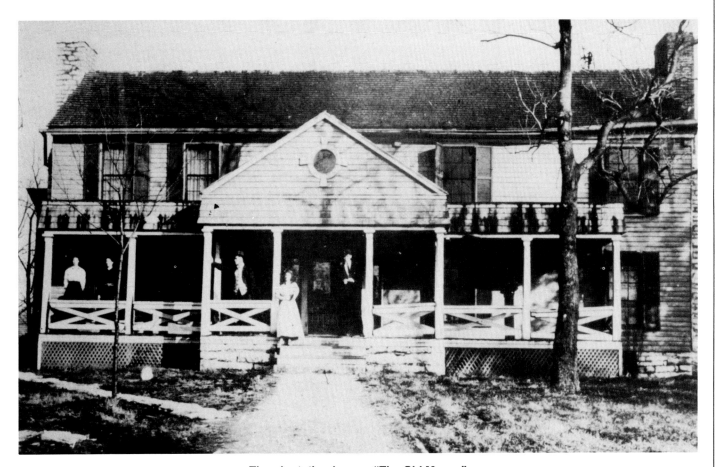

The plantation house, "The Old Manse"
The upper window at left looks out from what served as the first office of Madison College.
The room below it was the first classroom. (See related photograph on page 69.)

Madison College smoothly entered the 1940s but Dr. Sutherland, still directing for over forty years, sensed financial discomfort for the institution. Dr. Sutherland remained president until 1946 when he went to serve as the Secretary of the Association of Self-Supporting Institutions and Commission of Rural Living. He returned to Madison in his retirement.

Dr. Sutherland's intuition proved valid when the school entered the 1960s with a half-million dollar deficit and without any resources to pay its creditors. February 3rd, 1963 marked a drastic transition and reorganization after sixty years when a two-thirds majority voted that the operation of Madison College and Sanitarium join the Seventh-day Adventist Church under the Southern Union ownership. The hospital has since experienced extraordinary expansion and success.

The Seventh-day Adventist Church grew out of the worldwide mid-19th century religious revival and is today a mainstream Christian religion with approximately ten million members in two hundred countries. The church provides an array of humanitarian services around the world. In addition to healthcare services, it operates the world's largest Protestant school system and an international development and relief agency. Adventists manage 160 hospitals, 60 in the United States alone, as well as some 200 clinics and dispensaries around the world, all of which are committed to providing the finest health care in the spirit of compassion.

Since TCMC admitted its first patient in 1908, the hospital realized that total health care depends on a balance of physical, mental, social, and spiritual well-being. As the 21st century approaches, TCMC's commitment to providing outstanding facilities strengthens. It is equipped with a substantial inventory of high-tech diagnostic tools and treatments that serve the diverse needs of Nashville residents and surrounding areas. In addition to excellent services in the medical/surgical areas, TCMC provides various specialty services including emergency medicine, neurosurgery, cardiovascular, plastic, orthopaedic and laser surgery using advanced technology, to name a few. Its 18,000-square-foot comprehensive therapy center has a large pool, weight room, greenhouse, and rooms designed for rehabilitation and behavioral-related therapies. In partnership with Baptist Hospital, TCMC completed a five-story, 95,000 foot medical office building in 1996. The Baptist Medical Plaza at TCMC houses physician groups specializing in diverse areas and provides the very best in medical and surgical services.

TCMC continues to be a source of physical, emotional, and spiritual healing for those in need. Its physical rehabilitation services offer a comprehensive range of services to help those who have lost physical independence. A group of specialists representing essential disciplines, such as physical therapy, occupational therapy, recreational therapy, speech pathology and social services all work together to develop an effective rehabilitation plan that helps close the difference between goals and limitations.

The Center for Behavioral Medicine at TCMC offers mental health and chemical dependency treatment for seniors, adults, and teens. Tennessee Christian Counseling Centers offer a wide variety of counseling and outpatient therapy services. Each of TCMC's six area counseling centers—Madison, Portland, Murfreesboro, Franklin, Gallatin and Springfield—are staffed by experienced psychiatrists, clinical psychologists, licensed social workers and counselors providing treatment and support in individual, family, and group settings.

Sunbelt Home Health Services helps ease the transition from hospital to home and facilitates wellness and independence with personalized attention and patient education, faster recovery and help in healing. Home health care also provides the opportunity for family and friends to participate in patient care. Patients' spiritual needs are addressed as Chaplain Services are available for support during times of grief, loss, isolation, and adjustment to disabilities.

TCMC continues to be a place where the total needs of those being served are considered. The early beginnings of hard work and commitment are still felt today. Since its founding nearly 100 years ago, TCMC brings years of experience in clinical excellence, community education, and extraordinary patient care to a rapidly changing world. Today, the view that total health is a combination of physical, emotional, and spiritual wholeness and life is best when one enjoys good health is still at the core of its mission—a mission to "reflect the life and work of Christ and to assist physical, emotional and spiritual healing."

Services available at the Tennessee Christian Medical Center:

- Addiction treatment
  - Chemical dependency
  - Detox
  - Dual addictions
  - Intensive outpatient programs
  - Outpatient counseling
  - Partial hospitalization
- Anesthesiology
- Biofeedback
- Broncho-esophagology
- Cardiac catheterization
- Cardiovascular surgery
- Chemotherapy
- Clinical dietetics
- Colon/rectal surgery
- Comprehensive therapy center
- Critical care medicine
- Day surgery
- Dentistry
- Diabetes management
- Emergency medicine
- Endocrinology
- Endoscopy
- Enterostomal services
- Exercise testing
- Family medicine
- 55Plus Senior Club
- Fitness center
- Gastroenterology
- General surgery
- Gynecology
- Head and neck surgery
- Health education
- Health Information Resource Center
- Home health
- Internal medicine
- Laboratory services
- Laser surgery
- Lifeline
- Medical imaging
  - Angiography
  - Bone densitometry
  - Cardiac cath
  - CT
  - Echo cardiography
  - Mammography
  - MRI
  - Nuclear medicine
  - Stereotactic needle biopsy
  - Ultrasound
- Nephrology
- Neurology
- Neuropsychology
- Neurosurgery
- Obstetrics
- Occupational health
- Oncology
- Ophthalmology
- Oral surgery
- Orthopedics
- Pathology
- Pharmacy
- Physician referral service
- Plastic surgery
- Pre-admission testing
- Podiatry
- Psychiatry
  - Adolescent
  - Adult
  - Christian treatment
  - Geriatric
  - Outpatient counseling
  - Medical psychiatry
  - Partial hospitalization
- Pulmonary diseases
- Rehabilitation services
  - Occupational therapy
  - Physical therapy
  - Speech therapy
  - Recreation therapy
- Renal dialysis
- Same-day surgery
- Social services
- Subacute care
- Tennessee Christian Counseling Center
  - Outpatient therapy
  - Addiction treatment
  - Counseling
- Trauma Center, Level 2
- Urgent care
- Urology
- Volunteer services
- Wellness programs
- Women's diagnostic center
  - Bone density testing
  - Mammography
  - Stereotactic needle biopsy

VANDERBILT UNIVERSITY MEDICAL CENTER

Throughout its history, VUMC has combined the missions of patient care, medical and nursing education, and biomedical research for the benefit of the people of Middle Tennessee, the South, and the nation.

The Medical Center's precursor institution actually predates Commodore Cornelius Vanderbilt's gift that led to the establishment of a new university in Nashville. The Nashville Medical College, founded in 1850, merged into the new Vanderbilt University in 1874. Since those early days, when the entire school was housed in a building on Rutledge Hill, VUMC has grown to become an institution that has an impact on thousands of lives in Middle Tennessee and across the nation.

As an academic medical center, Vanderbilt University Medical Center offers many services that are unique to the region. Vanderbilt University Hospital, supported by research-based medical and nursing schools, delivers both routine inpatient care and highly specialized medical treatment and surgical procedures. The hospital is also home to the region's only Level 1 Trauma Center, Burn Center, Poison Control Center, and Liver Transplant Program. Its emergency air transport system, Life flight, has carried more than 8,500 patients to Vanderbilt and other hospitals in the past decade. Another important component of the Medical Center, the Vanderbilt Cancer Center, is one of 58 National Cancer Institute-designated cancer centers in the nation.

The Bill Wilkerson Center for Otolaryngology and Communications Sciences consolidated the private, not-for-profit Bill Wilkerson Center with Vanderbilt's Depart-

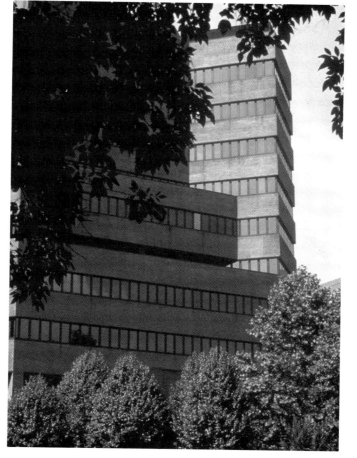

ment of Otolaryngology on July 1, 1997. This entity provides a new level of care to patients with otolaryngologic and communications diseases and disorders. The center is one of the nation's few communications disorders centers with expertise in clinical medicine, education, and research.

Vanderbilt Children's Hospital, designed to meet the special needs of children, provides comprehensive care for acute and chronic illnesses. The combined concentration on pediatric research, medical education, and patient care has led to many new techniques and discoveries. The hospital's pediatric trauma team is on call 24 hours a day. It operates specially equipped ambulances for the regional transport of high-risk newborns to the hospital, which has the area's only Level III neonatal intensive care unit.

The Vanderbilt Medical Group comprises more than 700 doctors and 95 outpatient specialty clinics, providing more general and specialty care than any other multi-specialty practice in the region. In addition to the customary specialties, VUMC offers more than 50 special centers and programs in areas such as addiction, arthritis, heart disease prevention, pediatric ophthalmology, pain control, balance and hearing disorders, and sports medicine, just to name a few.

In addition to its teaching role, Vanderbilt University Medical Center has a continued commitment to biomedical research. Research has been at the forefront of the center's mission for more than 70 years, and VUMC is one of the top 25 medical school recipients of research support from the National Institutes of Health. Through its research, VUMC has

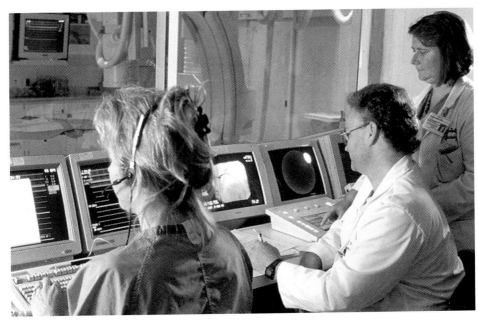

made medical advancements in the treatment of cancer, diabetes, cardiovascular disease, and many other diseases. NIH data shows that four basic science departments at VUMC now rank in the top seven nationally in attraction of total dollars of NIH support. Two Nobel prizes have been awarded to Vanderbilt professors. Earl W. Sutherland, Jr., M.D., professor of physiology, won the 1971 Prize for his discovery of "Cyclic AMP." The 1986 Nobel Prize in Physiology or Medicine (shared with Rita Levi-Montalcini) for the discovery of "Epidermal Growth Factor" was awarded to Stanley Cohen, Ph.D., American Cancer Society Research Fellow of Biochemistry.

All of these distinctions contribute to VUMC's repeated impressive showing in the *U.S. News & World Report* ranking of America's Best Hospitals. For example, in 1998, the Medical Center placed among the nation's top 50 health care institutions in seven specialties and among the top 20 in four. *U.S. News & World Report* also judged Vanderbilt University Hospital as the top hospital in Tennessee and ranked the Vanderbilt Medical School as number 15 among 125 medical schools nationwide. More than half of all the doctors in Nashville received at least part of their training at Vanderbilt, which also has one of the country's largest training programs for advanced nurse practitioners.

Aside from its academic and medical endeavors, VUMC is Nashville's largest private employer, with more than 8,500 people on its payroll. VUMC provides more than $40 million a year in uncompensated and charity care to patients. It generates more than $1.2 billion annually in local eco-

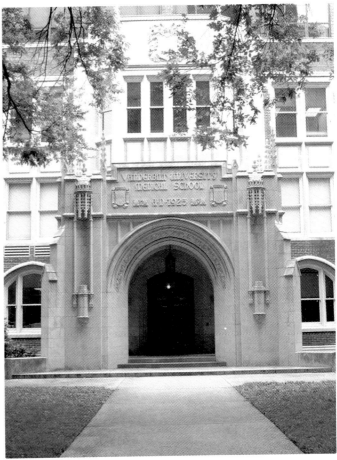

nomic activity. With its international reputation Vanderbilt University Medical Center is geographically, economically, and medically at the heart of Nashville and Middle Tennessee, always there to meet the medical needs of the region and beyond.

TENNESSEE ORTHOPAEDIC ALLIANCE

Tennessee Orthopaedic Alliance consists of 24 physicians— 23 orthopaedic surgeons and one physical medicine and rehabilitation specialist. Dr. Thomas E. Tompkins is the current president of Tennessee Orthopaedic Alliance. The Alliance physicians include Dave A. Alexander, M.D., John Bruno, III, M.D., Daniel S. Burrus, M.D., Mark R. Christofersen, M.D., Philip G. Coogan, M.D., William M. Gavigan, M.D., Jeffrey L. Herring, M.D., Stanley G. Hopp, M.D., David S. Jones, M.D., E. Ray Lowery, M.D., J. Wills Oglesby, M.D., Daniel L. Phillips, M.D., Eugene M. Regen, Jr., M.D., Richard A. Rogers, M.D., Barrett F. Rosen, M.D., James L. Rungee, M.D., Robert V. Russell, M.D., Stuart E. Smith, M.D., Gray C. Stahlman, M.D., Catherine R. Stallworth, M.D., Robert E. Stein, M.D., Stewart F. Stowers, M.D., Thomas E. Tompkins, M.D., and Roderick A. Vaughan, M.D.

Tennessee Orthopaedic Alliance began in 1926 and 1932 with the pioneering practices of Dr. George K. Carpenter, Sr. and Dr. Eugene M. Regen, Sr. Dr. Carpenter started the practice that would become Nashville Orthopaedic Associates and Dr. Regen founded Orthopaedic Surgical Associates.

Dr. Carpenter was a graduate of Vanderbilt University. He completed both pediatric and orthopaedic training, the latter from Massachusetts General Hospital in Boston and Hillman Hospital in Birmingham, Alabama. After World War II, Dr. Carpenter established a preceptorship program in orthopaedic surgery. He trained many orthopaedic surgeons before they returned to private practice.

In 1947 Dr. Carpenter invited Dr. S. Benjamin Fowler to join his practice. Dr. Fowler received medical training at the University of Tennessee and completed his orthopaedic training at the Orthopaedic Hospital of Los Angeles, Los Angeles, California. Dr. Fowler achieved international acclaim in hand and general orthopaedic surgery. He was the Founding Member and President of the American Society for Surgery of the Hand (1955) and President of the American Academy of Orthopaedic Surgeons (1969-70).

Don L. Eyler, M.D., Thomas F. Parrish, M.D., and Charles M. Hamilton, M.D. joined Drs. Carpenter and Fowler to form Nashville Orthopaedic Associates. With the addition of Drs. Fowler and Eyler, the orthopaedic preceptorship program became a hand fellowship and trained both national and international orthopaedic surgeons.

Eugene M. Regen, Sr., M.D., was the sixth orthopaedic surgeon in Nashville and began his practice in 1932. Dr. Regen graduated from Vanderbilt University and trained in orthopaedics at both Vanderbilt University School of Medicine, Nashville, Tennessee, and at Cleveland City Hospital, Cleveland, Ohio.

Dr. Regen, whose first love was teaching, was instrumental in establishing the Department of Orthopaedic Surgery at Vanderbilt School of Medicine and was clinical professor of Orthopaedic Surgery at Vanderbilt. He retired in 1981 after 50 years of teaching and practice.

In 1994 Nashville Orthopaedic Associates merged with Orthopaedic Surgical Associates to form Tennessee Orthopaedic Associates. Tennessee Orthopaedic Associates continued to grow in both size and geographic extent with the addition of Orthopaedic Specialists of Murfreesboro in 1996.

In October, 1996 Tennessee Orthopaedic Associates joined with The Lipscomb Clinic to form Tennessee Orthopaedic Alliance. At the same time, this newly-formed group became a founding practice in OrthoLink Physicians Corporation. Ortho-Link is a physician-crafted, physician-directed practice management company that provides its affiliated practices the resources and infrastructure necessary to compete in the evolving healthcare marketplace.

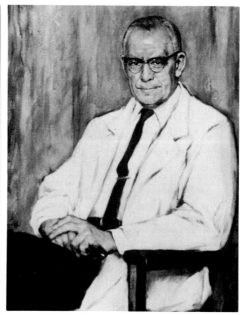

George K. Carpenter, Sr., M.D.   Eugene M. Regen, Sr., M.D.

BIBLIOGRAPHY

BOOKS

Harriette Simpson Arnow, *Flowering of the Cumberland.* New York: Macmillan, 1963

_____, *Seedtime on the Cumberland.* New York: Macmillan, 1960

Paul K. Conkin, *Gone With the Ivy; A Biography of Vanderbilt University.* Knoxville: The University of Tennessee Press, 1985

Robert E. Corlew, ed., *Tennessee; A Short History.* Second edition. Knoxville: The University of Tennessee Press, 1981

Alfred Leland Crabb, *Nashville; Personality of a City.* Indianapolis: Bobbs Merrill, 1960

H, W. Crew, *History of Nashville, Tennessee.* Nashville: Publishing House of the Methodist Episcopal Church, South, 1890. Reprinted by Charles Elder Bookseller, n.d., 1972

Don H. Doyle, *Nashville Since the 1920s.* Knoxville: The University of Tennessee Press, 1985

Daniel Drake, *Practical Essays on Medical Education, and the Medical Profession in the United States.* Reprinted: Cincinnati: Roff and Young, 1932

Walter Durham, *Nashville; The Occupied City; The First Seventeen Months. February 16, 1862 to June 30, 1863.* Nashville: Tennessee Historical Society, 1985

_____, *Reluctant Partners; Nashville and the Union; July 1, 1863 to June 30, 1865.* Nashville: Tennessee Historical Society, 1987

Anita Shafer Goodstein, *Nashville 1780-1860; From Frontier to City.* Gainesville: The University of Florida Press, 1989

Philip M. Hamer, *The Centennial History of the Tennessee State Medical Association.* Nashville: the Association, 1930

Timothy Jacobson, *Making Medical Doctors; Science and Medicine at Vanderbilt Since Flexner.* Tuscaloosa: University of Alabama Press, 1987

Rudolph H. Kampmeier, *History of the Tennessee Medical Association, 1930-1980.* Nashville: the Association, 1981

_____, *Recollections, The Department of Medicine, Vanderbilt University School of Medicine, 1925-1959.* Nashville: Vanderbilt University Press, 1980

Howard A. Kelly, *A Cyclopedia of American Medical Biography, Compiling the Lives of Eminent Deceased Physicians and Surgeons from 1610 to 1910.* Two Volumes. Philadelphia: W. B. Saunders, 1912

Magali Sarfatti Larson, *The Rise of Professionalism; A Sociological Analysis.* Berkeley: University of California, 1977

Roderick E. McGrew, *Encyclopedia of Medical History.* New York: McGraw-Hill, 1985

Henry McRaven, *Nashville; "Athens of the South."* Chapel Hill: Scheer and Jervis, 1949

Samuel Riven, *The Road South.* Nashville: The Association for Tennessee History, 1993

William G. Rothstein, *American Physicians in the Nineteenth Century; From Sects to Science.* Baltimore: Johns Hopkins Press, 1972

Ronald N. Satz, *Tennessee's Indian People; From White Contact to Removal, 1540-1840.* Knoxville: The University of Tennessee Press, 1979

Henry Burnell Shafer, *The American Medical Profession, 1783-1850.* New York: Columbia University Press, 1936

Richard Harrison Shryock, *The Development of Modern Medicine.* New York: Alfred A. Knopf, 1947

Robert G. Spinney, *World War II in Nashville: Transformation of the Home Front.* Knoxville: The University of Tennessee Press, 1998

Paul Starr, *The Social Transformation of American Medicine.* New York: Basic Books, 1982

James Summerville, *Educating Black Doctors; A History of Meharry Medical College.* Tuscaloosa: The University of Alabama Press, 1983

William Waller, editor, *Nashville, 1900 to 1910.* Nashville: Vanderbilt University Press, 1972

ARTICLES

Murray C. Brown, "Venereal Disease Case Reporting as Protection to the Physician-Patient Relationship," *Journal of the Tennessee State Medical Association,* 37, no. 1 (January, 1944)

John C. Burch, "Functions of County Societies," *Journal of the Tennessee State Medical Association,* 45, no. 5 (May, 1947)

Kyle C. Copenhaver, "Medical Practice in Tennessee," *Journal of the Tennessee State Medical Association,* 38, no. 5 (May, 1945)

James X. Corgan, "Notes on Tennessee's Pioneer Scientists," *Journal of the Tennessee Academy of Science,* 53, no. 1 (January, 1978)

Paul DeWitt, "Some Observations on the Selective Service System," *Journal of the Tennessee State Medical Association,* 12, no. 5 (September, 1919)

J. L. Farringer, Jr., "A History of Hospitals in Davidson County, Tennessee," *Journal of the Tennessee Medical Association,* 67, no. 4 (April, 1974)

Robert M. Foote, "Growth of Specialized Programs for Tennessee Children," *Journal of the Tennessee State Medical Association*, 45, no. 11 (November, 1952)

V.O. Foster, "The Physician and School Health," *Journal of the Tennessee State Medical Association*, 41, no. 2 (February, 1948)

R. H. Hutcheson and C. B. Tucker, "Doctors of Medicine Registered in Tennessee; A Distribution of Physicians," *Journal of the Tennessee State Medical Association*, 43, no. 1 (January, 1950)

W. S. Leathers, "Some Significant Achievements in Public Health," *Journal of the Tennessee State Medical Association*, 35, no. 12 (December, 1942)

J. T. Moore, Sr., "Brief Review of Therapeutic Measures During the Last 53 Years," *Journal of the Tennessee State Medical Association*, 45, no. 11 (November, 1952)

"Report of the Committee on Prepayment Plans for Hospital and Medical Services," *Journal of the Tennessee State Medical Association*, 36, no. 10 (October, 1943)

N. S. Shofner, "The Tennessee Plan," *Journal of the Tennessee State Medical Association*, 43, no. 3 (April, 1950)

H. H. Shoulders, "State Medicine," *Journal of the Tennessee State Medical Association*, 29, no. 1 (January, 1936)

Daugh W. Smith, "Medicine's Place in Society," *Journal of the Tennessee State Medical Association*, 45, no. 4 (April, 1952)

_____, "Shall We Coast Now—Or Forge Ahead?" *Journal of the Tennessee State Medical Association*, 46, no. 4 (April, 1953)

W. C. Williams, "Tennessee's State Health Program," *Journal of the Tennessee State Medical Association*, 29, no. 5 (May, 1936)

Otis S. Warr, "Medical Education in Tennessee; An Historical Sketch," *Journal of the Tennessee State Medical Association*, 23, no 8 (August, 1930)

Olin D. West, "A Discussion of the Reports of the Committee on the Costs of Medical Care," *Journal of the Tennessee State Medical Association, 26*, no. 6 (June, 1933)

W. H. Witt, "The Progress of Internal Medicine Since 1830," in Philip M. Hamer, *The Centennial History of the Tennessee State Medical Association*. Nashville: the Association, 1930

UNPUBLISHED MATERIALS

James Summerville, "Organized Medicine in Nashville; The First Century, 1821-1921," M.A. thesis, Vanderbilt University, 1983

John B. Thomison, "The History of Medicine in Nashville." Available at Historical Collections, Eskind Biomedical Sciences Library, Vanderbilt University School of Medicine

INDEX

GENERAL

Italicized page numbers indicate an illustration

22, 25-27, 40; in civic life of early Nashville, 23-24; public standing of, 22, 23, 24, 27; competition among, after Civil War, 49, 53, 55; lack of therapeutic consensus among, 14, 22, 25, 50, 53, 54; rise of specialization among, 53; relationship of, with sectarians, 53, 56; professional unification of 57; seek public health reforms, 59-62, 65; and the American Medical Association, 62, 64; growing political strength of, 64-65; economic advancement of, 22-23, 41, 49, 71; in the Great War (World War I), 87; rising public expectations of, 89-90; and the New Deal, 91, 95; and Tennessee Department of Public Health, 91-94; political stances of, 1930s-1960, 90-94, 107-108; in World War II, 97-98, 111; competition among, in modern times, 123

Physicians, Tennessee: censuses of, 20, 71

Plunket, James D., *51*, 54

Porter, Robert M., 42

Price, George H., *45*, 61

Protestant Hospital, 85. *See also* Baptist Hospital

Public health. *See various headings under* Nashville

Public Health Department, Nashville, 99, 100

Public Health Department, Tennessee, 91-92

Pure food and drug laws, 60-62

R

Ramsey, Frank A., 20

Red Cross, 97, *99*

Richards, A. Frank, 88, 91

Ricketson, Greer, 89

Riven, Samuel, 98, 101

Roane, James, 21, 22, 24

Roberts, Deering J., 62

Robertson, Felix, 8, 11, 15, 22, 24

Robertson, James, *8*, 11

Robinson, Canby, *46*

Ruger, Ferdinand, 19

Rush, Benjamin, 10, 11, 13

S

Sappington, John, 11

Sappington, Mark, 14

Satcher, David, 112

School health programs, 95

Science, in antebellum Tennessee, 19

Sell, Sarah H., *125*

Sevier, John, 10

Shadden, L. L.

Shelby, John, 15, 43

Shelby Medical College, 43-44

Shoulders, Harrison, 84, 91, 92, 102

Smith, Daugh W., 101, 103, 108

Smith, Larkin, 61

Sneed, William J., 47

Southern Hills Medical Center, 6,118

Stout, Samuel, 29-31, 35

Southern Practitioner, 62

St. John's Hospital, 73

St. Margarete's Hospital, *84*

St. Thomas Hospital, 81-84, *96, 101, 106*, 118

St. Vincent's Hospital, 73

Stahlman, Mildred, 118

Stewart, Ferdinand A., 69

Summers, Thomas O., Jr., 41

Summit Medical Center, 118

Surgery: in early Nashville, 11, 21-22; in post-Civil War city, 53; rising place of, 84;

first open-heart, in Tennessee, *106*

Sutherland, Earl, 111

Swift, Ebenezer, 33

T

TennCare, 122-23

Tennessee Christian Medical Center, 69

Tennessee Hospital, 76

Tennessee Medical Association: wins passage of physician licensing law, 55-56; growth of, in early 20th century, 64; and Nashville Academy of Medicine, 65, 102; offers continuing education, 89; public service campaigns of, 93-95; creates prepaid health insurance plan, 108; establishes malpractice insurance company, 125

Thayer Veterans Hospital, *102*, 103

Thomison, John B., 11, 89, *125*

Thompson, John R., 105, 108

Thomson, Samuel, 17

Thomsonian system, 17-18

Townsend, Arthur M., 70

Trabue, Charles C., IV, *94*, 101, 103, 113, 117

Transylvania University, *21*, 23

Trawick, Arch M., 57

Troost, Gerard, 19

Tuberculosis, 59, 104

Tucker, Newton G., 56

Turner, Edward L., 111

Typhoid, 59, 62

U

University of Nashville: medical department, 18, 24, 27, 31-32, *42*-43; merges

with University of Tennessee medical department, 44-45; and Flexner Report, 66-67

University of Pennsylvania, medical school at, 15, 18, 27

University of Tennessee medical department, *45-46*, 66-67, 76, 78

V

Vanderbilt University School of Medicine, *45-46*, 67, 76, 97-98, 109-111

Venereal disease, 34, 98-99

Volunteer State Medical Association, 69

W

Walker, Matthew, 105, 112

Walker, William, *26*

Waters, John, 22, 23

Watson, John M., *31*, 42

Wesley, John, 16, 17

West, Harold D., 111, *112*

West, Olin, 62, 90, *91*

Whitacre, Frank, 88

White, James, 11, 14

White, John, 34

White, G. R., 60

Williams, Daniel Hale, 76-77

Williams, W. C., 92

Wilson, John Robertson, 22

Winchester, E., 11

Winston, Charles K., 23, 27, 39, 42

Witherspoon, John A., *45*, 60, 62

Women in Nashville medicine, 64, 124, *125*

Woodring, Thomas, 25

Y

Yandell, David W., 29

Yandell, Wilson, 25

Youmans, John, 46, 97, 101, 109, *110*